D1373725

THE PICTURE
OF HEALTH

ALSO BY ERIK P. ECKHOLM

Losing Ground
Environmental Stress and World Food Prospects

THE PICTURE
OF HEALTH

Environmental Sources of Disease

ERIK P. ECKHOLM

WORLDWATCH INSTITUTE, WITH THE SUPPORT AND
COOPERATION OF THE UNITED NATIONS ENVIRONMENT PROGRAM

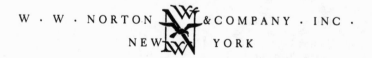

W · W · NORTON & COMPANY · INC ·
NEW YORK

Copyright © 1977 by Worldwatch Institute
Published simultaneously in Canada by George J. McLeod Limited,
Toronto. Printed in the United States of America.
All Rights Reserved
First Edition

Library of Congress Cataloging in Publication Data
Eckholm, Eric P
    The picture of health.
    Bibliography: p.
    Includes index.
    1. Environmental health. 2. Social
medicine. 3. Nutritionally induced diseases.
I. Worldwatch Institute. II. United Nations.
Environment Programme. III. Title.
RA565.E4   362.1'042   77-11896
ISBN 0-393-06434-4

1 2 3 4 5 6 7 8 9 0

Contents

Foreword by Mostafa K. Tolba 7

Preface 11

1. Ways of Life, Ways of Death 17

2. The Picture of Health Today 21

3. The Human Geography of Undernutrition 38

4. Mutinous Bounty: Hazards of the Affluent Diet 63

5. Cancer: A Social Disease 89

6. The Unnatural History of Tobacco 113

7. Something in the Air 133

8. Who Pays for Production? 154

9. Of Snails and Men 174

10. The Family Planning Factor 189

11. Creating Better Health 206

Notes 222

Suggested Readings 245

Index 247

Foreword

BY DR. MOSTAFA K. TOLBA,

Executive Director, United Nations Environment Program

I n 1972, the General Assembly of the United Nations unanimously recognized "the need for prompt and effective implementation by governments and the international community of measures designed to safeguard and enhance the environment for the benefit of present and future generations of man." To this end, the General Assembly established the United Nations Environment Program.

At its first meeting in Geneva in June 1973, the Governing Council of UNEP declared its intention "to provide, through interdisciplinary study of natural and manmade ecological systems, improved knowledge for integrated and rational management of the resources of the biosphere, and for safeguarding human well-being as well as ecosystems."

In keeping with its broad concern for the enhancement of environmental quality, and above all because of the imperative of satisfying basic human needs, UNEP is devoting considerable attention to the study and amelioration of environmental threats to human health. Thus, UNEP has been concerned with, for example, controlling endemic diseases, monitoring pollution and studying its health effects, establishing an International Register of Potentially Toxic Chemicals, developing environmentally sound pest-management systems, and controlling cancer caused by environmental intervention.

These and related initiatives have as their long-term purpose the better management of human activities so as to protect the human environment. If the goal of better environmental management is to be achieved, we must create a climate of public awareness about the dangers that a badly managed environment can create for human health and well-being, and thus a willingness to support measures designed to avoid those dangers.

Therefore, UNEP fully supports the Worldwatch Institute in its efforts to draw public attention to the global threats to human health and well-being. It is natural for UNEP to support the preparation and publication of this book, although the views expressed here remain, of course, the exclusive responsibility of the author.

The Picture of Health deals comprehensively and in a readable manner with many of the environmental factors that endanger the attainment and maintenance of health, a condition that the World Health Organization has defined as "a state of complete physical, mental and social well-being." This book should interest and assist government officials, medical and health practitioners, scientists involved in health issues, and laymen. Its carefully chosen references provide a basis for further reading for those who choose to delve deeper into the realms of environmental health.

Many of the health hazards described in this book may strike some as being of interest mainly to the richer countries, but the time may not be far off when developing nations, too, will have to give more attention to these problems. Developing countries have the advantage of being able to learn from the experience and mistakes of others. Meanwhile, they have to cope with formidable environmental health problems of their own. The extreme case of schistosomiasis, which is discussed in this book, is a case in point.

Those concerned with health problems in developing countries are faced with a vast interlocking set of challenges.

More particularly, inadequately met human needs for food, shelter, clothing and education serve to compound the basic health problem. For developing countries the prime necessity is for further development, but of a sort that pays due regard to environmental conditions and that can be sustained over the long term.

With all the pitfalls the path to perfect health involves, people can probably count themselves fortunate if they die, as his biographer claims Wordsworth did, "of nothing serious." Perhaps this book and similar efforts will help us move toward a world in which such an epitaph applies to all.

Preface

While I have tried in this book to review the major environmental influences on health today, I make no claim of comprehensiveness. The subject is as broad as one wants it to be and, in striving to write a readable, up-to-date, and accurate book, I have had to omit—often reluctantly—discussion of many relevant issues. The massive problems of, for instance, mental health, alcoholism, and accidents are not examined. I do feel, however, that all the topics discussed are crucial ones, and that most of the more important omitted topics are covered implicitly in my general conclusions. Because this book is about disease causes and their prevention rather than disease treatment, medical-care strategies (as opposed to preventive health strategies) receive little attention.

Those who find this book useful are indebted (as I am) to Frank Record, whose energetic research efforts provided a solid foundation for the analysis of health problems. Frank also contributed substantially to the discussion of the affluent diet in Chapter 4. With her deft editorial hand, Kathleen Courrier helped to clarify, economize, and enliven my prose. Blondeen Duhaney's cheerful efficiency made the production of the manuscript a far less painful task than it might have been. Marion Frayman also chipped in at critical times with much-appreciated secretarial assistance. The supporting research that Sandy Callier and John Sanders carried out in Latin America proved quite valuable.

Either in person or by mail, hundreds of individuals around the world generously contributed their ideas and papers as our research proceeded. But I am especially grateful to the dozens of men and women who took time to read through my early drafts, point out errors, and suggest improvements. The entire manuscript was reviewed by: Dr. O. Alozie, UNEP; Lester Brown, Worldwatch Institute; Dr. B. H. Dietrich, World Health Organization; Dr. René Dubos, Rockefeller University; Dr. Sándor Eckhardt, National Institute of Oncology, Budapest; Dr. Hugh de Glanville, *Medicine Digest;* Dr. D. J. Jussawalla, Tata Memorial Hospital, Bombay; Dr. John H. Knowles, Rockefeller Foundation; Dr. Philip R. Lee, University of California at San Francisco; Dr. N. P. Napalkov, Petrov Research Institute, Leningrad; Linda Starke, Worldwatch Institute; Jon Tinker, Earthscan, London; and Dr. A. Olufemi Williams, University of Ibadan.

The following individuals reviewed portions of the manuscript dealing with their special areas of expertise: Dr. Aaron M. Altschul, Georgetown University; Dr. Nicholas A. Ashford, Massachusetts Institute of Technology; Dr. Alan Berg, World Bank; Dr. John W. Berg, University of Iowa; Dr. Denis P. Burkitt, Medical Research Council, London; Barry Castleman; Dr. John Cooper, National Cancer Institute; Dr. Jaoquín Cravioto, Institucion Mexicana de Asistencia a la Niñez; Dr. Joseph F. Fraumeni, Jr., National Cancer Institute; Dr. Gio B. Gori, National Cancer Institute; Davidson Gwatkin, Ford Foundation; Dr. William Haenszel, National Cancer Institute; Dr. John Higginson, International Agency for Research on Cancer; Dr. M. J. Hill, Bacterial Metabolism Research Laboratory, London; Dr. Andrea M. Hricko, University of California at Berkeley; Dr. Junichi Iwai, Brookhaven National Laboratory; Dr. Michael Jacobson, Center for Science in the Public Interest; Dr. J. S. Lehman, Jr., Edna McConnell Clark Foundation; Dr. W. F. Miner, U. S. Naval Medical Research Unit, Cairo; Dr. Robert Morris; Dr. Phyllis

Piotrow, Population Crisis Committee; Dr. Jon E. Rhode, Gadja Mada University, Jogjakarta; Dr. Patricia Rosenfield, Resources for the Future; Dr. Jesse Roth, National Institutes of Health; Sheldon W. Samuels, AFL-CIO; Dr. Nevin S. Scrimshaw, Massachusetts Institute of Technology; Dr. Mitsuo Segi, Segi Institute of Cancer Epidemiology, Nagoya; Dr. Irving J. Selikoff, Mount Sinai Medical Center, New York; Dr. Eugene Seskin, Resources for the Future; Michael Sharpston, World Bank; Dr. J. J. Speidel, Agency for International Development; Dr. Carl E. Taylor, Johns Hopkins University; and Dr. Christopher Tietze, Population Council.

Most of Chapter 6 appeared in the April, 1977, issue of *Natural History.* Much of Chapters 3 and 4 appeared in *The Two Faces of Malnutrition* (Worldwatch Paper 9, December 1976), written with Frank Record. Parts of Chapter 10 appeared in *Health: The Family Planning Factor* (Worldwatch Paper 10, January 1977), written with Kathleen Newland.

Special thanks are due the United Nations Environment Program for financing the bulk of our research on environment and health. I am particularly grateful to Dr. Mostafa K. Tolba, UNEP's Executive Director, for his strong personal support for this project; and to Alastair Matheson, Chief of Communications, who coordinated UNEP's expert review of the manuscript. Finally, the general support given Worldwatch Institute by the Rockefeller Brothers Fund, the Edna McConnell Clark Foundation, and Robert O. Anderson has enabled the Institute to cosponsor projects of this type and to build its public-education capacity. Naturally, responsibility for the book's contents remains mine alone.

ERIK P. ECKHOLM
Worldwatch Institute

*1776 Massachusetts Ave., N.W.
Washington, D. C. 20036*

THE PICTURE
OF HEALTH

1. Ways of Life, Ways of Death

THE DAY before her forty-fifth birthday, a New Jersey woman learns that she is dying. The lining of her chest cavity has been invaded by cancer. Her doctor is puzzled: he has seen this rare malignancy only in asbestos workers, and this patient is a lawyer. But as he sifts through the records of her past, the origins of her tragedy become clear. The patient's father had spent 1947 working in an asbestos-insulation factory. His clothes and hair had been covered with whitish fibers when he came home from work each evening, and his daughter had frequently laundered his work clothes. The father, like tens of thousands of former asbestos workers around the world, died of cancer two decades after his stint in the factory. Now, still another decade later, the daughter discovers that her own fate was sealed thirty years ago.

The parents of a three-year-old Ecuadorian girl watch helplessly as chronic diarrhea takes her life. They are unaware that in lands where everyone has access to clean water and where children are well nourished, diarrhea seldom takes lives. Nor do they know that their daughter is but one of thirty-five thousand small children who die every day, in many cases because undernutrition has sapped the victims' ability to survive simple infectious diseases. As the parents compare the straggly crops on their eroded patch of hillside with the lush hacienda fields below, they do realize that, unlike the family of the hacienda owner, their remaining-five children will be kept from sleep by hunger.

Widowed at age forty-two by her husband's heart attack, an Englishwoman doubles her devotion to her eighteen-year-old son. More than devotion will be necessary, however, if a similar catastrophe is not to strike the son when he reaches middle age; the family's rich diet is promoting deadly arterial degeneration. The son, who smokes as much as his father did, has a vague fear of developing lung cancer in old age. He does not suspect that cigarettes, like fatty foods, contributed to his father's sudden demise—and are helping to lay the groundwork for his own heart attack. Both mother and son would be surprised to learn that one in three of their acquaintances—indeed, one in three people in North America and Europe—will succumb to heart disease.

Alongside the River Nile, a *fellah*, or peasant farmer, plants his second cotton crop of the year. His government has dammed the river upstream and now the irrigation canals carry water year-round. As he stoops to pull a weed, he is wrenched by pains in his lower abdomen and he feels unusually tired; once again he will be unable to finish his day's work. As he relieves himself on the canal bank, he unwittingly returns to the water thousands of parasite eggs in his urine, which has turned blood-red. The fellah's plight is not his alone. While year-round irrigation has boosted incomes in his village, half the villagers now complain of internal pains and fatigue. Three have died of inexplicable causes. Like 200 million others who live near slow-moving tropical waters and lack safe sewage facilities, he is infected with schistosomiasis.

Individuals who enjoy good health rightly think of themselves as fortunate. But luck has little to do with the broad patterns of disease and mortality that prevail in each society. The striking variations in health conditions among countries and cultural groups reflect differences in social and physical environments. And increasingly, the forces that shape health patterns are set in motion by human activities and decisions. Indeed, in creating its way of life, each society creates its way of death.

The "environment" that influences health involves much more than the esthetic state of our natural surroundings with which many associate the term. Social and economic policies that leave people too poor to purchase adequate diets, without access to safe water, or ignorant of the rudiments of sanitation all affect health. So do production processes and political decisions that permit the pollution of workplaces or neighborhoods with dangerous substances. Individuals' eating, drinking, smoking, and exercise habits form the roots of many major diseases; and these habits are in turn influenced by cultural traditions, economic institutions, and governmental policies.

Given particular environmental conditions, health patterns within societies can thus be predicted. Where undernutrition and filth reign, infectious diseases and childhood deaths are commonplace. Overeating, sedentary living, and smoking take their toll among the middle-aged in the forms of cardiovascular diseases and cancer. Where industry is not closely regulated, workers in mines, factories, and fields often pay, through job-induced disease and death, an extraordinary price that never figures into production costs.

The ideal of a disease-free existence for all may never be realized. Humans are evolving, disease agents are evolving, and the biological, geological, and chemical features of the environment are changing faster than ever as humans lend an unskilled hand. Still, by making effective use of what we know about the sources of ill health, we could vastly reduce unnecessary suffering and the frequency of premature deaths.

Major improvements in health will not be achieved, however, by pouring more and more funds into costly curative

measures. Changes in the social structures and personal behavior patterns that promote diseases will do far more than
doctors and drugs can to minimize the burden of disease and
the tragedy of early death. Better health may require, for
instance, land reforms in El Salvador, the control of air pollution in Japan, and well-digging programs in rural India; dietary changes in the United States, a cut in cigarette smoking
in Scotland, and the control of cotton dusts in an Egyptian
textile factory.

Identifying environmental threats to health is, of course,
far easier than overcoming them. Unlike advanced medical
technologies, the social changes essential to better health
cannot usually be purchased, lent, or donated. An inquiry
into environmental influences on health involves delving
into economics, politics, personal lifestyles, and humans' relationships with their natural surroundings. The picture of
health is, ultimately, a reflected image of society.

2. The Picture of Health Today

THE GLOBAL PICTURE of health cannot be sketched in a few simple strokes. As big as life, the subject is largely invisible. Few statistics on the frequency of nonfatal illnesses exist, though it is in terms of their lifetime disease experiences that most people would characterize their own health. The expansive definition of health nobly inscribed in the charter of the World Health Organization—"a state of complete physical, mental and social well-being"—is beyond the ken of statisticians and even stumps philosophers. Almost inevitably, students of "health" trends wind up studying the causes and frequency of death. Mortality data give an admittedly incomplete picture of the health scene; but death is what statisticians like to call a "clearly defined event," and every country tries to keep track of the ways its citizens die.

One common measure of health conditions is life expectancy at birth. In 1975, the world's average newborn could expect to live about fifty-nine years.[1] But a country-by-country comparison of life spans reveals that place of birth all too often determines age at death. Infants born in the more desperately poor countries of Africa have a life expectancy of only about forty, while life expectancy in the world's more developed countries has now passed the Biblical ideal of three score and ten.

In a scattering of Asia's poorest countries—Bangladesh,

Nepal, Laos, and others—and in many sub-Saharan African
countries, life is often short, if not brutal. Life-expectancy
averages in these nations hover below forty-five, mainly because so many die in infancy or childhood. Where deaths
among the young are common, the national life-expectancy
average is, of course, low even though many of those surviving childhood may live to ripe old ages. With average life
spans close to fifty, Indians and Pakistanis are slightly better
off; their life expectancy at birth is comparable to that which
prevailed in the United States and Great Britain in 1900.
Reliable data on health trends among the 800 million Chinese are not to be had, but some credible estimates put
Chinese life expectancy at about sixty-two years.

Average longevity in most other Asian countries and in
the Middle East generally ranges from fifty to seventy years.
Latin American and Caribbean countries show the most consistently high national averages among the "less developed"
regions, with life expectancies generally topping sixty. Yet
even in the Western Hemisphere, people in a few of the
poorest countries—including Haiti, Guatemala, Nicaragua,
and Honduras—have average life spans of under fifty-five
years.

Infant mortality rates are another useful measure of
health. Reflecting deaths among babies before they reach
their first birthdays, infant mortality may be a more sensitive
indicator of social and health conditions than life-expectancy
averages are. Infants and small children are especially hard
hit by inadequate food supplies, poor sanitation, and deficient medical care. Sweden boasts the world's lowest infant
mortality rate. Only nine of every thousand Swedish babies
die before reaching age one. Infant mortality in other more
developed countries around the world ranges between ten
and twenty-five deaths per thousand live births. Put otherwise, only one or two of every hundred babies in these countries dies within a year of birth. In contrast, one in thirteen

babies in Latin America; one in seven babies on the Indian subcontinent; and one in five babies in parts of Africa dies by age one.[2]

The international disparities in the survival odds of both infants and small children bespeak the most drastic difference in the health plights of the poor and the rich. In most poor countries, deaths among children under five occur with soul-numbing frequency; in many cases they account for more than half of all deaths. In parts of Latin America, observes nutritionist Alan Berg, "the making and selling of minicaskets are common sights." In more developed countries, fewer than 5 percent of all deaths strike infants and small children.[3]

Internationally, longevity correlates roughly with per capita income levels. Nearly all societies with average life spans above seventy years have average personal incomes above a thousand dollars a year; in most of them, personal incomes average several thousand dollars. People with life expectancies below fifty earn on average no more than a few hundred dollars annually. Still, finer comparisons of incomes and mortality rates around the world prove that national wealth doesn't always determine national health.

In some countries, national life-expectancy averages range far higher than income levels would suggest. In 1975, newborn Cubans could expect to reach their 70th birthdays, though their annual per capita income was only $540. Even more surprising, the average Sri Lankan had a life expectancy of sixty-eight years and an annual income of only $200. Against these examples may be juxtaposed that of Brazil, where average life expectancy was only sixty-one years despite an average personal income of $750 per year, and Libya, where an oil-bloated per capita income of about $3,000 belied an average life span of fifty-three. Such comparisons reveal that income and social-service distribution within countries critically influence national health conditions. The data from Cuba, Sri Lanka, and elsewhere also show that if certain nutritional, sanitary, and health-care needs are met, the relatively poor can enjoy excellent health. Apparently, people need not be as rich as the Swiss to be fit as the Swiss.

Poorer people or regions within countries, like poorer countries internationally, tend to have the highest infant mortality rates and the lowest life-expectancy averages. For example, while the more affluent classes in Brazil or Mexico share health standards with Finns or Canadians, some of the landless rural residents of these countries face mortality odds comparable to those faced by people in far poorer countries. But—further proof that glib generalizations about income and health don't hold—the average income in the Indian state of Kerala is among the lowest in the nation, yet Kerala's rural infant mortality rate is well below half the Indian national average. And, at sixty-one years, the life expectancy there is well above the national average. Along with land reforms, the mass distribution of educational programs, food subsidies, and health services has improved the health of Kerala's residents dramatically in spite of their penury.[4]

Income levels, economic and social discrimination, or differences in lifestyles often affect the health of cultural or ethnic subgroups. Nonwhites in the United States, for example, tend to die younger than whites do. On the other hand, members of the Seventh-Day Adventist Church, who consume a low-fat, meatless diet and eschew tobacco and alcohol, suffer far less heart disease and cancer than the average American does. In the United States and elsewhere, better-educated people generally outlive the poorly educated.[5]

Because of the wide disparity in the average life spans of men and women, years of widowhood are the inevitable lot of most married women. For both biological and social reasons, women tend to outlive men; moreover, as health conditions improve, the gap in life spans between the sexes widens. In the more affluent countries, females outlive males by six to eight years. Living habits partially explain this gap: men are more apt than women to smoke, to drink heavily, to commit suicide, and to be exposed to toxic substances on the job. They are also more likely to die in automobile crashes and at the hands of murderers. But women also appear genetically destined to survive their male contemporaries. In particular, fewer women than men suffer heart attacks in midlife.

Although statistics from India, Pakistan, and a few other Asian and African countries seem to contradict the global pattern, data usually show that females outlive males in poor countries too. The sex-related differences in longevity are less spectacular than they are in richer countries, however. The special burden borne by millions of low-income women —decades of childbearing in a context of poor nutrition and inadequate sanitation—robs them of part of their inherited health advantage. In some cultures, another part is sacrificed to the family tradition of discriminating against female children in the allotment of food supplies, education, and other benefits.[6]

Causes, as well as rates, of death differ radically between the poor and the rich. The leading killers in poor countries are the infectious diseases—dysentery, pneumonia, tuberculosis, bronchitis, influenza, measles, and so forth—that ravaged Europe and North America less than a century ago. Often bolstered by undernutrition, infections take an especially large toll among small children in poor countries. Although less susceptible than children to the effects of either undernutrition or infection, poor adults are more likely than affluent ones to die from any of scores of infectious diseases. They are also susceptible to a multitude of dangerous parasites and, like adults everywhere, to heart diseases and cancer.

Infections (above all the common cold) still plague the affluent, but relatively few of the rich die from infection.

Accidents claim far more children's lives than any diseases do in rich nations. Over time, mortality in developed countries has come increasingly to reflect the presence of just two categories of noninfectious diseases—cardiovascular ailments and cancer. Responsible for about half of all deaths in the industrial countries, cardiovascular diseases are by a considerable margin the major disease problem in these nations and are the leading cause of death among middle-aged men and older people of both sexes. Cancer, which claims roughly a fifth of all lives in the industrial countries, ranks second as a health challenge. While it mainly victimizes the aged, cancer often strikes younger people; and in some countries it now leads all other diseases as a killer of children.

At the height of the empire, Romans lived an average of about thirty years each. As recently as the 1930s, life expectancy at birth in Africa, Asia, and Latin America averaged an estimated thirty-two years as well. But throughout most of the developing world in the fifteen years that followed World War II, mortality rates fell and life expectancy climbed with a speed unmatched in European or North American history. Average life expectancy at birth in the developing countries has now topped fifty years.[7]

The steep climb in life expectancy in developing countries occurred in the era of modern medicine, but most analysts grant little credit for the progress to health-care measures per se. True, DDT has cleared malaria from some regions, and a vaccine sounded smallpox's death knell; moreover, antibiotics have undeniably aided the treatment of some infections. Yet, modern medical technology has touched the lives of so few people that its advent can scarcely have wrought such dramatic health improvements. Instead, more general economic and social changes have probably driven down premature mortality among the poor, just as they did in the late nineteenth and early twentieth centuries

in Europe and North America.⁸ For example, better nutrition—a product of agricultural progress and of better transportation and communications—has undoubtedly reduced
mortality rates. Improved water supplies and sanitary facilities have also proved life-savers. An indefinable "modernization" process that has involved the spread of education, the
radio, and modern ideas about personal hygiene has left its
mark on health as well. Perhaps most significant, economic
development—however unequally apportioned—has raised
the incomes and altered the worldviews of billions of people.

Whatever the relative contributions of medical care and
other social changes to postwar health improvements, the
period of quick gains in the health status of the poor may now
be over. In its *Fifth Report on the World Health Situation,*
published in 1975, the World Health Organization stated: "It
seems that after the rapid drop in mortality observed between 1950 and 1960 a 'consolidation' period is needed and
that a further decline in mortality will depend on conditions
largely beyond the control of the health sector."⁹ What are
these unmet essential preconditions of better health? A review of the underlying causes of disease and death in developing countries provides the answer.

Undernutrition, infections spread via human excrement,
and airborne infections together form what Michael Sharpston of the World Bank has termed "the basic disease pattern
of poverty." These three types of diseases normally account
for 70–90 percent of all childhood deaths in poor countries.
While the relative importance of particular categories and
diseases varies from one low-income area to another, their
combined impact varies little and is "rooted in the ecology
of poverty."¹⁰

Diets deficient in calories, protein, or other essential nutrients kill some people outright. But the chronic undernutrition that plagues at least several hundred million people
takes far more lives indirectly as an accomplice of infectious

diseases. An unholy alliance between undernutrition and infections accounts largely for the frequency of infant and
childhood deaths today and must thus be regarded as the
world's single most menacing health problem.

While nutrition influences personal susceptibility to and
the severity of infectious diseases, sanitary conditions usually
determine the frequency with which people come into contact with disease-causing bacteria, viruses, and parasites.
Where household and community hygiene is lax, disease
agents can proliferate wantonly. Even when water and sewage facilities are close at hand, individuals who do not understand sanitation's impact on good health cannot be expected
to use them regularly enough to control disease. Moreover,
when the only available potable water must be head-carried
several kilometers (a task usually relegated to females) or
must be purchased at high prices with scarce family funds,
little will be used for washing cooking utensils, hands, and
clothes. And when sewage treatment or disposal is haphaz-
ard, water supplies, soil, and the home may be invisibly contaminated with human excrement and its dangerous cargo of
infectious agents.

Drinking and cooking water must be reasonably germ-
free to be reasonably safe. But, field studies consistently
show, once water meets a certain minimum standard, the
quantity of water readily available to families influences
their health even more than the water's purity does—a re-
flection of the exceptional health importance of water for
cleanliness.[11]

Although water-supply engineers have been hard-
pressed to keep up with booming populations, the proportion of the world's people living near safe and abundant
water has increased fairly steadily since midcentury. The
number of people who still lack such access, however, remains scandalously large. Analyzing the situation as of 1975
in all the developing countries except China, the World

Health Organization (WHO) estimated that 1.2 billion people, or 62 percent of developing country residents, lived without adequate water supplies. Rural people are especially deprived; four-fifths of them, as opposed to a fourth of urban residents, lacked easy access to safe water.[12]

To make a bad story worse, many municipal water systems in Africa, Asia, and Latin America (and also in some developed countries) provide water of unreliable quality. Urban water systems are often contaminated when illegal hook-ups are made or when huge variations in water pressure allow polluted groundwater to seep into the pipes. According to a recent WHO survey, the urban water systems in most developing countries are not even inspected properly for biological contamination.[13]

The global sewage scene looks even bleaker than the water economy. One of the most dangerous substances to which people are commonly exposed, untreated excrement well deserves the low social esteem in which it is generally held. The disease and death traceable to environmental pollution by human excrement dwarfs the known toll taken by industrial pollutants. Raw sewage is the principal conveyor of the intestinal infections (such as diarrhea, cholera, and typhoid) that collectively constitute a leading cause of death in countries that together contain two-thirds of the world's people.

Careless handling of human wastes also spreads debilitating parasites. Yet in 1975 two-thirds of those in the developing countries (excepting China)—about 1.4 billion people—lacked access to safe latrines or sewage systems. A fourth of the urban and almost nine-tenths of the rural populations of these developing nations lived without this health necessity.[14]

Where hunger and filth mar daily life, modern medicine cannot work health miracles. To be sure, certain applications of medical technology, especially immunizations, pay off

dramatically anywhere. For example, smallpox, an age-old
purveyor of death and disfigurement, may well be eradicated
altogether in 1977 or soon after as a result of the World
Health Organization's international campaign. Only a decade ago, smallpox ravaged much of Africa, Asia, and Latin
America, and returned sporadically to developed countries
as well.[15]

A triumph of medical science and international cooperation the smallpox program has been; but a watershed in
health history it is not. The core disease pattern of poverty
will not be defeated by medical technology alone. A manifestation of extreme economic deprivation, undernutrition will
bow only to economic reforms. Sanitary conditions will pass
muster only where governments invest heavily in water-
supply and waste-disposal facilities and where personal
cleanliness becomes normative.

Even as smallpox has been conquered, another classic
scourge, cholera, has reared up with a vengeance. A dreaded
plague of nineteenth century Europe, cholera was for
decades thought to have been driven back into its South
Asian homeland for good. Since 1961, however, cholera has
embarked for the seventh time in recorded history on a
deadly intercontinental march—this time from a base in Indonesia. The disease now claims victims all over Asia and the
Middle East and in much of Africa. Cholera spreads from
person to person via sewage and impure water and food, and
health officials fear that an infected traveler may soon introduce the blight to Latin America, where poor sanitation
would give it wide scope.[16]

Armed with DDT, health officials once dreamed of exter-
minating malaria, a major threat to life throughout Africa
and parts of Asia and Latin America. Malaria-bearing mosquitoes, however, have proved far more tenacious than was
once thought. Since World War II, control programs have
freed large areas of Asia, Latin America, and the Mediterra-

nean region from malaria, but the disease is now staging a comeback in some of the freed zones. In sub-Saharan Africa, where the disease was never suppressed, malaria still kills a million children every year. Several mosquito strains have now become immune to DDT and other low-cost pesticides, and hopes for a malaria-free planet have been quietly shelved.[17]

Malaria numbers among a host of parasitic diseases that people in poor countries must contend with on top of their heavy burden of bacterial and viral infections. Two other less well known parasitic diseases—schistosomiasis and filariasis —rival malaria in the staggering number of people they affect; like malaria, each now infects at least 200 million people, as many as inhabit the United States. The number of lives debilitated or cut short by both schistosomiasis and filariasis grows steadily because of human recklessness or neglect. The schistosomiasis parasite passes from person to person by way of body wastes and waterborne snails, and the massive present-day construction of reservoirs and irrigation canals in countries lacking proper sewage control creates ever more new habitats for the parasite. Similarly, a type of mosquito-spread filariasis is gaining ground in the overflowing slums that ring most poor-country cities; there, the culprit mosquito species breeds in clogged open drains and in standing pools of sewage-polluted water.[18]

Malaria, schistosomiasis, filariasis, and three other so-called tropical diseases (trypanosomiasis, leprosy, and leishmaniasis) are the targets of a major new international program of research and prevention. And well they should be. Whereas an explosive increase in basic biomedical knowledge since World War II has revolutionized many aspects of medical care in the industrialized countries, the World Health Organization notes, "these advances have as yet hardly begun to be applied to the problems of tropical disease," for which "methods of control and treatment have scarcely changed in the past thirty years." Announcing the new program in late 1975, WHO estimated that the total global research budget for all tropical diseases in that year amounted to only about $30 million—less than one-twentieth of the amount spent on cancer studies alone.[19]

Medical research priorities do indeed need to be shifted toward the diseases of the poor. But no scientific breakthroughs can conquer these afflictions if the ecological conditions that promote them persist. After all, many of today's "tropical" diseases once blighted life in temperate, now-developed countries too. In 1793 in Philadelphia, which was then the United States' capital, mosquito-borne yellow fever caused what has been called "the greatest single disaster ever to befall an American city." In a single year, some 13,000 people—a third of the population—fled the city; most of those remaining fell ill, and more than 4,000 people died.[20] Malaria was also a major health threat in southern Europe and in the southern United States early in the current century. Many "tropical" diseases could easily thrive in temperate latitudes again if public-health and sanitation measures were to break down.

In developed countries, infections and undernutrition have gradually loosened their stranglehold. Other death-dealing syndromes, the so-called degenerative diseases, now claim far more lives in rich countries. Foremost among these is coronary heart disease (the familiar heart attack), the cause of about one-third of all deaths in most affluent nations. Heart attacks, strokes, and cancer together cause two-thirds of all deaths in North America, Europe, and the more developed East Asian countries.[21] Not since the plague decimated Europe have so few diseases accounted for such a high proportion of deaths over large areas.

Cardiovascular diseases and cancer have been labeled "degenerative" because human susceptibility to them seems to rise with age. But in some ways the label is misleading. Far from the inevitable onslaught of old age, many deaths in developed countries are premature. No one can say how long the average human is biologically programmed to live in the absence of negative environmental influences. But available evidence proves that cardiovascular and cancer rates among the affluent, like infection rates among the poor, reflect people's habits and habitats. Each year, "degenerative" diseases kill hundreds of thousands who have not yet lived three score and ten years.

While personal genetic endowments undoubtedly stack the cards, dietary excesses, sedentary lifestyles, and cigarette smoking all seem to promote heart attacks and other cardiovascular diseases. Competitive and stressful living, some recent research shows, may also shorten life. Largely because of coronary heart disease, *overall* mortality rates among men between the ages of about fifty and seventy have actually increased in several developed countries since 1950. For men in late middle age, the relatively new risk of heart disease has risen, while the old danger from infectious diseases has stopped declining. According to data from affluent countries on three continents, from 50 to 60 percent of all coronary deaths take those under age seventy-five; and from 15 to 25 percent of these deaths involve people under fifty-five.[22]

Taking into account the huge international and intercultural variations in cancer patterns, most scientists aver that some 70 to 90 percent of all cancer can be blamed on environmental causes. Many cancer sources remain undiscovered, but some are known and others are under strong suspicion: tobacco smoke, various dietary factors, ultraviolet and ionizing radiation, and assorted industrial chemicals and pollutants head the list of untouchables. Since most cancer has environmental rather than genetic origins, most cancer could, theoretically, be avoided. And since 65–80 percent of all cancer deaths in many developed countries strike people younger than seventy-five, and 15 to 25 percent strike people under age fifty-five, cancer cannot simply be dismissed as a "degenerative" disease of old age.[23]

Lifestyles and other environmental influences in developed countries have been linked to many other leading causes of death besides cardiovascular diseases and cancer. The fast-climbing incidence of diabetes is apparently affected by a combination of genetic and dietary factors. Cirrhosis of the liver usually stems from alcoholism. Emphysema and chronic-bronchitis rates are unquestionably boosted by cigarette smoking and urban air pollution. Accidents, suicides, and homicides obviously have social origins.

When the health scenes in richer and poorer countries are compared, some striking symmetries appear. Whereas undernutrition often kills the poor, overnutrition—resulting from high calorie and fat intakes—has emerged as a medical scourge among Europeans and North Americans. Like undernutrition, overnutrition reduces life expectancy, increases susceptibility to disease, and reduces productivity. While the affluent seldom need fear the biological contamination of their water supplies, they cannot help but worry about the possible presence of disease-causing metals and carcinogenic chemicals in their water. The smoke of wood or dung cooking-fires, which sullies the air that the world's poorest half breathes, rarely reaches the nostrils of the rich; but both tobacco smoke and air poisoned by auto and industrial pollutants do.

All available evidence indicates that personal behavior patterns—especially smoking, dietary habits, drinking, and lack of exercise—are the major sources of premature death in developed countries today. Yet, as any newspaper reader in these countries can attest, another kind of health threat has emerged as well. With growing frequency we read of modern environmental-health catastrophes: a rash of cancers among the workers in an American factory; a cloud of lethal chemicals settling over an Italian community; an outbreak of cancer among women whose mothers took certain drugs during pregnancy. Diseases unleashed in workplaces, by pollution, or by misuses of technology may be inadvertently caused, but only the ingenuous can regard them as accidental. The frequency and predictability with which they occur show that some diseases are built into present-day industrial society. Those concerned about the conservation of natural beauty have long demanded that technological and economic decisions be suffused with an environmental ethic. Today, rudimentary knowledge of what abused technology can do to human health provides an even stronger rationale for social change.

The Japanese, as physically cramped as they are industrially advanced, have probably suffered more "manufactured" diseases than have any other people. In 1970, Japan's "economic density," the ratio of its economic output to its usable land, was more than eleven times that of the United States.[24] And, until recently, the welcome noise of incredibly rapid industrial growth in Japan drowned out the warnings of ecologists.

The mercury-poisoned people of Minamata, whose sin was to eat fish from Minamata Bay, have become a worldwide symbol of pollution-caused health disaster. Hundreds, maybe thousands, of people in Minamata and elsewhere in Japan have been tormented or killed by an incurable disorder of the central nervous system that warps both the body and the mind. Hapless Japanese have also been the first mass victims of cadmium poisoning. Several hundred cases of itai-itai (literally, "ouch-ouch") disease, so named because of the cries its victims release as their bones disintegrate, have been identified in the Jinzu River basin, where soils and waters are laced with the cadmium wastes of upstream mines and smelters.[25]

Well-publicized environmental-health scares such as that

in Minamata, London's deadly air-pollution episode in 1953, or the accidental release of a poisonous chemical cloud over Seveso, Italy, in July of 1976, only hint at a problem of unknown dimensions. Such disasters are recognized only when concentrations of a poison are so great or affect an identifiable group of people for so long that marked health damages occur. But even as major pollution tragedies, industrial "accidents," and fatal toxic exposures inside factories make headlines, residents in more developed regions routinely eat, drink, and breathe extremely low levels of a multitude of unnatural materials. Some of the substances that have infiltrated modern life—lead, asbestos, and PCBs (polychlorinated biphenyls) to name a few—are known to be dangerous; countless others have unknown effects. Moreover, the long-term effects of breathing in or ingesting minute quantities of common pollutants, individually or together, have not been determined.[26]

The residents of modern industrial societies live in a chemical environment without historical precedent, an environment filled with traces of substances that have never before contributed to the evolution of species. The unhealthy influence of the foul air that shrouds many cities is well established; but, apart from that, no widespread health damage has yet been directly linked to chronic, low-level exposures to the metals, industrial chemicals, pesticide residues, and other agents that permeate daily life in industrial countries. Quite possibly, no such damage will ever be proven—either because most of these agents actually are harmless or because the damages they cause may be too subtle and various to detect. Carcinogens often take decades to wreak their damage, and deleterious genetic mutations may not reveal themselves for generations; such time lapses make neat cause-and-effect arguments about the impact of carcinogens or mutagens on health extraordinarily difficult to frame. To say that massive eco-catastrophes are definitely in the works is almost as foolish as saying that none could occur. No one knows what is in store—but unquestionably, the reckless handling of technology and industrial growth boosts the likelihood that human-caused diseases will be unleashed.

The ailments normally associated with affluence and industrialization are not confined to developed countries. Many wealthier urbanites in even the poorest countries smoke, overeat, and underexercise—and they suffer accordingly. Where few industries exist and where markets are not glutted with space-age concoctions, widespread chemical contamination is unlikely; but, on the other hand, African, Asian, and Latin American governments are less likely than those in Europe and North America to have the resources to regulate working conditions inside and pollution levels outside the industries that do exist in their countries. Then, too, the automobile has brought to the sidewalks of many poor-country cities air pollution that does not discriminate among its victims by income levels. Dangerous pesticides, sometimes imported from countries where their use is banned, are often applied by farmworkers who have no idea of the hazards such use poses.

In terms of health, at least, no group is more luckless than the unknown number who now face simultaneously the health risks of their own poverty and of other people's wealth. Lacking adequate food, housing, and water supplies, they are ready victims of infectious diseases and parasites; but they must also contend with the toxic effluents of affluence. To be strapped by the health hazards but shorn of the comforts of modern industrial society is to be poor indeed.

3. The Human Geography of Undernutrition

THE "WORLD food crisis" has recently become headline-caliber news. Aspects of this "crisis," however, have quietly haunted the back pages for decades. The world food problem actually comprises numerous components, some old as civilization, some new as the 1970s, all intermeshed, but each analytically distinct.

One aspect of the food problem that always rivets public attention is famine. Modern communications, trade, and aid all help check the local starvation that regional crop failures once heralded. But even today when the harvest fails in destitute or isolated areas, or when war disrupts food production and trade, famine may clench its bony fist.

No image more effectively conjures a Malthusian nightmare among the well-fed majority than that of the gaunt faces of the starving. Yet famine, however horrid and however photogenic, is in every case a localized disaster whose impact can be warded off, sometimes entirely, by effective national and international planning. However, the measures essential to forestall famines—early detection and aid—will not combat other crucial components of the food problem.

Disruptions in the world's commercial food market since 1972 have probably generated even more public anxiety worldwide than has famine. As the global demand for food outstripped available supplies, reserves were drawn dangerously low, prices multiplied as they never had before, and food-surplus countries imposed unprecedented controls on food exports. Events demonstrated graphically that the comfortable surpluses and stability of the postwar global food market can no longer be taken for granted.

The horror of recent famines and the jolt of tripling grain prices have diverted attention from the most basic and widespread food problem of all: the chronic undernutrition suffered by the world's poor. Undernutrition is an invisible crisis, a daily tragedy that deprives hundreds of millions of the right to realize their genetic potential—their birthright. Pervasive and lasting, undernutrition does not make dramatic news copy, but its toll in human life far outweighs that of occasional famines.

The various components of the world's food problem are, of course, closely interconnected. Developments in one profoundly affect those in another. When grain reserves run low, for example, the international capacity to stave off imminent famines with food aid shrinks commensurately. As grain prices soar, so does the number of undernourished people. Those spending 60–80 percent of their income on food, as hundreds of millions do, can hardly offset a doubling in the price of grain by spending more.

But though undernutrition is intertwined with the commercial food market's crisis of supply, demand, and management, the two problems are not identical. Widespread undernutrition predated the food-market turbulence of the 1970s and, should government policies stabilize the food market, will outlast the storm. Even if our reserve bins overflow again, undernutrition will still have a firm hold. A manifestation of poverty, undernutrition has roots in the political and economic structures that engender economic deprivation— roots that will not be totally eradicated by wise planning alone, but only through fundamental social and institutional reform.

In any specific case, dietary deficiencies may be tied to various "causes." As victims of ignorance and superstition, people sometimes fail to use indigenous foods wisely. Or, impressed by advertisers and the examples set by wealthier women, mothers may switch their nursing infants from breast to bottle even though adequate quantities of commercial infant formulas are beyond their financial reach. Overcrowding resulting from population increases, inequitable land distribution, or both, leaves some rural families without enough land to grow the food they need. Others are left landless.

Each of the many factors linked to undernutrition is in some sense a manifestation of poverty. The poor, wherever they live, are susceptible to undernutrition; the rich everywhere can purchase an adequate diet. The persistence of widespread undernutrition in a world that produces ample food for all can only be construed as a measure of the failure of the global social order.

Perceptions of the scale and severity of undernutrition in the world have changed along with our data-gathering methods and our understanding of human dietary needs. The United Nations estimates of the protein requirements of a healthy person, for example, were scaled downward by about a third in the early 1970s. But some recent studies suggest that the redefined protein standards may be too low; a group of U.S. university students fed the new "safe" level of protein developed signs of protein deficiency after two months. On the other hand, those raised on a protein-rich diet may come physiologically to require more protein than those accustomed to a lower-protein diet.[1]

A related shift in scientific thinking stems from the understanding of how protein and food energy interact in the body. Both are essential for body growth and maintenance, but when the body is short of calories, available protein is poorly utilized and may be burned as energy to make up the deficit. Thus, even though a patient may show overt signs of a protein shortage, the underlying problem may be more complex—a deficiency of energy, or protein, or both. (In view of these possible protein-energy interactions, doctors commonly use the general term "protein-calorie malnutrition" to describe the undernutrition of the poor.)

From 1950 to 1970, official estimates of the extent of undernutrition in the world fell steadily. No one can say how much of the drop reflected true nutritional gains, and how much reflected changing definitions and improved statistical methods. All three factors probably came into play.

Researchers in the U.N. Food and Agriculture Organization and the U.S. Department of Agriculture who conducted several global surveys in the first three decades after World War II reached the same conclusion: close to half of humanity suffered from shortages of protein or calories or both. All these estimates, however, were based on questionable assumptions about consumption needs, and most relied on national food-consumption averages that ignored subnational variations in food habits and income. In preparation for the 1974 World Food Conference, the United Nations reassessed the world nutrition situation using the latest notions of nutritional requirements and, for the first time, considering rich as well as poor countries. This study showed that 460 million people—or one of every six people included in the survey— were undernourished as of 1970.[2]

Unfortunately, the U.N. study could not include data on China, North Korea, and what was then North Vietnam, but most observers feel that severe undernutrition is probably rare in these societies. Some suggest that these latest U.N. estimates still overstate the problem, especially as it exists in Africa and the Near East. On the other hand, the canvassers claim that they used a quite restrictive notion of adequate nutrition and that "a less conservative definition might give a much higher figure" for the number of undernourished. Furthermore, the years of the survey—1969 through 1971—were years of generally good weather, high production, and low food prices. Large jumps in food prices nearly everywhere in subsequent years have undoubtedly pushed people who were formerly on the borders of undernutrition into that unhappy state.

Whatever the exact number, hundreds of millions of people are simply not getting enough food to lead active, healthy lives. Some in this group suffer from undernutrition so extreme that it threatens their existence directly. Community examinations show that at any given time about 1 to 7 percent of the preschool children in poor countries weigh less than 60 percent of their expected weights—a desperate condition akin to walking death.[3] Among this exceptionally deprived minority of children, the vicious and potentially fatal diseases of severe undernutrition are apt to appear: the protein-deficiency disease kwashiorkor, characterized by bloated bellies, wasted muscles, and apathy; and marasmus, which results from gross shortages of energy and protein and leaves its victims looking like little more than bags of bones and skin.

Severe undernutrition mainly strikes small children, who need about twice as much protein and energy per pound of body weight as adults require. Pregnant and nursing mothers, who also need extra food, form a second nutritionally vulnerable group. In many cultures, small children and females of all ages are discriminated against in the allocation of family food supplies, which makes these two groups all the more vulnerable.

The severely undernourished, those close to starvation, probably number in the tens rather than the hundreds of millions. While a far cry from the stereotyped notion that "half the world is starving to death," this number is still unconscionably large. When they do not starve, these victims of the modern economic order face the possibility of living with irreversibly stunted bodies and minds. And, clinical surveys reveal, significant, if less dramatic, undernutrition affects as many as half to two-thirds of the children in poor countries.[4] Even when undernutrition is not directly lethal, it raises the odds of early death from other causes. At the least, it impairs health and infringes upon the right to a full life.

Besides energy and protein shortages, the problem of undernutrition encompasses numerous specific vitamin and mineral deficiencies that usually coexist with overall underfeeding.[5] By far the most widespread of these is anemia, a condition often resulting from inadequate intake of iron or other vitamins or from iron losses to blood parasites like hookworm. Widespread in all countries, anemia afflicts 5 to 15 percent of all adult men and even higher proportions of women and children in many regions. Anemia saps the energy needed to work and raises a person's susceptibility to disease; it also multiplies a woman's chances of dying during childbirth.

Vitamin A deficiencies rank as the leading cause of childhood blindness in many developing countries. Xerophthalmia (literally, "dry eye") is the general term for ocular disorders brought on by vitamin A shortages, disorders that range from an inability to see in dim light to total blindness. A tenth of India's children are said to suffer "night blindness," and between 20,000 and 100,000 children around the world lose their sight completely every year for want of vitamin A.

Geographic comparisons of the scale of protein-calorie undernutrition are necessarily imprecise; the quality and kinds of information available vary considerably from one country to another. Nevertheless, available data show that most of the world's undernourished live in Asia. The densely populated and desperately poor countries of the Indian sub-continent—India, Pakistan, and Bangladesh—are especially hard hit. There, more people live in destitution and on less land than in any other large region, and vast numbers stave off nutritional disaster only until the inevitable failure of the monsoon every several years. Unpublished dietary surveys of India commissioned by UNICEF in 1974 reveal the sorry dietary plight of more than a third of all Indians. Some 224 million of India's 600 million people consume less than three-fourths of the calories they need, while fifty-three million of them take in less than half their minimum daily energy requirements.[6]

A generation back, China also teemed with the under-nourished and the outright starving. None of the hundreds of scientists, journalists, and doctors visiting China in the last few years, however, has reported observing any of the clinical signs of undernutrition that once blighted Chinese life.[7] China has not suppressed undernutrition by making great national gains in per capita food production, but rather by distributing food more equitably.

Africa has not yet reached the extremes of population density seen in parts of Asia such as Java or Bangladesh. But since unrelieved poverty is endemic, since modern agricultural techniques are rarely used, and since the farming potential of large areas is limited, undernutrition is widespread there. The recent lengthy drought in the Sahelian zone, just south of the Sahara, shocked the world into recognizing the threat of periodic famine that imperils many Africans. By the tens of millions, however, others also struggle unnoticed against chronic food shortages. About 30 percent of sub-Saharan Africa's children, calculates the World Health Organization, do not get the nutrients they need. Another 4 percent suffer severe, directly life-threatening undernutrition.[8]

Personal incomes throughout most of Latin America average considerably higher than those in most of Asia and Africa. Drastic disparities in income and access to farmland, however, have given undernutrition a long leash among the poor. According to the Pan American Health Organization (PAHO), from about 10 to 30 percent of the children in most Latin American countries suffer at least moderate undernutrition. Nutritional deficiencies are most common in Northeast Brazil, the Andes Mountains, parts of Central America and the Caribbean, and other places where economic exploitation and poverty are the harshest. Haiti, with its deadly trinity of extreme population density, accelerating soil erosion, and exceptional income disparity, has one of the world's highest rates of severe undernutrition among children.[9]

Oddly enough, little more is known about the prevalence of undernutrition in many rich than in many poor countries. In wealthy nations, generally high incomes and more or less adequate social welfare programs prevent much of the serious protein-calorie malnutrition of the sort rampant in the developing nations. Yet even in a country as rich as the United States, millions live in dire need and some live so far outside the mainstream of national life that government aid programs never reach them.

Available surveys of the nutritional state of Americans leave a basic question unanswered: How many are undernourished? Current investigations reveal that minor mineral and vitamin deficiencies are found throughout the populace. But studies conducted over the last decade have proved that more serious undernutrition plagues the American poor, especially Indians living on reservations, migrant workers, the rural poor, and the aged.[10] Well-publicized journeys by national political leaders into zones of deep poverty in the late 1960s exposed the entire nation to people with the vacant stares and underdeveloped bodies that are a common legacy of the undernourished poor everywhere. Subsequent publicity prompted the establishment of new programs designed to meet the basic food needs of the poor. But, clearly, even in a country where obesity is the leading nutritional disorder, economic deprivation and nutritional ignorance can exact their customary nutritional costs.

Deaths overtly due to underconsumption are uncommon. But the far broader and more insidious effects of nutritional deficiencies on human well-being are not. Simply put, deficient diets increase the frequency and intensify the effects of many other health problems. Lack of adequate amounts or of the right kinds of food is now strongly implicated as the principal cause of the inordinately high mortality among children in poor countries.[11]

By far the most extensive and reliable investigation of childhood mortality in the developing world, one that examined deaths among young children in fifteen regions in the Americas, was that published by PAHO in 1973. This study showed that nutritional deficiencies or infant immaturity (which includes both premature births and underweight births) were the *primary* causes of only 6 percent of deaths among children under five. However, nutritional deficiencies or immaturity were found to be *associated* with 57 percent of all child deaths.[12] Undernutrition thus probably contributes to more than half of all child deaths in Latin America; a comparable calculation in South Asia or Central Africa would likely yield an even higher figure.

As the numerous deaths associated with immature births imply, undernutrition can injure the unborn child. Underweight babies are especially susceptible to infections, and this frailty sometimes persists for many months. The exact impact of maternal nutrition on birth weights has not been well established, but evidence suggests that the influence begins long before a child is even conceived. In fact, the childhood diet of the mother, which helped determine her physical size and overall health, usually affects the newborn's

size. When a mother has been undernourished and unhealthy during her childhood, writes Dr. Herbert G. Birch,
"her pregnancy is more frequently disturbed and her child
more often of low birth-weight."[13] Undernutrition among
girls today thus imperils the health of the next generation.

Less surprising, studies have also revealed that the infant,
as well as the mother, can be harmed by dietary deficiencies
during the mother's pregnancy, especially when the mother
has a history of undernutrition. Nutritionists in Guatemala
who provided food supplements to pregnant women in two
villages found that the average birth weights of babies born
to the women increased by 9 percent over the prestudy
average. A research group working in another Guatemalan
village discovered that "contrary to the belief that the developing infant could successfully parasitize the mother for
whatever nutrients were needed for growth, . . . newborns
in the village are not normal—they are small at birth . . . and
nearly 20 percent show evidence of subtle intrauterine infection."[14]

Of all deaths among children under age five covered in
the PAHO study, nearly four-fifths struck infants in their first
year of life. The riskiest day for the newborn is the first, and
it is in the earliest days of life that the threats associated with
underweight birth hold most force. Then, in the following
months and years, infection and malnutrition interact with a
vengeance wherever conditions allow.

Limited and impure water supplies, inadequate sanitary
facilities and habits, and substandard housing together expose youngsters in developing countries to a host of infectious agents. Forty-five Guatemalan babies who were studied
during the first three years of their lives together suffered
nearly 2,500 episodes of infectious disease during that brief
period—an average of one disease every three weeks per
infant.[15] Weakened by poor nutrition, children living in unsanitary conditions succumb to the infectious agents ubiqui-

tous in their environment much more often than they would if they were properly fed. And when they do fall ill, the undernourished are far more likely than better-fed children to suffer severely. Diseases considered routine in more developed regions—diarrhea, measles, or chickenpox—are a routine cause of death among the poor.

Before the recent large-scale use of vaccine in many countries, measles afflicted children virtually everywhere. Yet, while fatalities from measles have long been rare in developed countries, death rates among those contracting measles in poor regions are sometimes as high as 15 percent. In some years, the fatality rate among children infected with measles in Mexico is 180 times higher than that in the United States, and the fatality rate in Ecuador is 480 times the U.S. rate. All evidence indicts nutritional factors as the primary cause of these radical disparities, and international comparisons of death rates from several other infections—among them whooping cough, tuberculosis, and diarrhea—reveal similar disparities.[16]

Even as undernutrition aggravates disease, infections may place nutritional stress on those whose diets would otherwise be barely adequate. Gastrointestinal infections reduce the body's ability to extract nutrients from food; and, even more significant, nearly all infections trigger the increased elimination of protein nitrogen through body wastes. Moreover, well-meaning parents often put children with gastrointestinal problems on diets less nutritious than usual in accordance with unfounded notions about which foods the sick should eat. Well-fed children can easily replace the nutrients lost to infection, but children living on the margins of malnutrition may never make up the deficit.

Most deaths associated with infant undernutrition occur during or after weaning, as mother's milk is supplemented with or replaced by other foods. The foods substituted for mother's milk during this critical period frequently fail to meet the child's nutritional needs. As leading nutritionists Nevin Scrimshaw and Moisés Béhar observe, the mortality rate of children from one to four years of age—those in the postweaning period—is the best measure of malnutrition in a country.[17] In more developed regions, only about one death occurs per thousand children aged one to four. In some of the poorest areas, forty or fifty deaths per thousand children occur—most of which better diets could prevent.

The interaction of all the threats associated with weaning, undernutrition, and poor sanitation are illustrated most forcefully by the problem of diarrhea. Those in well-nourished countries, for whom diarrhea is usually no more than an occasional nuisance brought on by impure food or forays into a foreign cuisine, may shudder to learn that diarrhea is a major worldwide killer. The upper respiratory infections together known as the common cold cause more discomfort than any other known disease, but diarrhea far outranks the cold as a cause of death.

Diarrhea takes children's lives in all countries, but its death toll in affluent areas is small today. In contrast, in many poorer countries, deaths from diarrhea (concentrated among children) outnumber those from any other cause. Nothing about this dismal picture is historically unique. At the beginning of the current century, children in Western Europe and North America succumbed to diarrhea at rates even higher than those of the poorest countries today. But improved diets and sanitation have left their mark, pushing down diarrhea-caused death rates for young children in developed countries to less than a hundredth of their past levels.[18]

Stressing the vulnerability of the young child, physicians have adopted the term "weanling diarrhea" to describe this deleterious syndrome. Diarrhea may strike a child any time after birth and is especially common in infants born underweight, but its frequency escalates radically during the weaning period. Exposure to unsterile foods and containers is inevitable once it becomes necessary to supplement mother's milk, and an increasingly mobile infant is an increasingly exposed infant. In developing countries, few babies between the ages of six months and two years escape diarrhea, and many suffer repeated episodes.

The trend toward premature abandonment of breast feeding in the swelling cities of Africa, Asia, and Latin America is boosting the frequency and severity of weanling diarrhea. Bottle feeding in an unsanitary milieu raises the odds that the infant will be exposed to infection; and when parents cannot afford proper substitutes for nutritious breast milk, the poorly nourished infant's resistance to disease decreases. The identification of bottle feeding with "modernity," the aggressive corporate promotion of infant formulas, the failure of employers to provide nursing facilities for working mothers, and even the donation of dried milk to poor families by well-meaning international aid agencies have all contributed to the dangerous shift from breast to bottle among the world's poor.[19]

Unsanitary living conditions and personal habits also promote weanling diarrhea. The bacteria and viruses that apparently cause diarrhea are passed from person to person through fecally contaminated food, water, and utensils, or, perhaps most often, from hand to mouth. But nutrition influences the ailment's severity. Among the better-off, diarrhea usually causes a few days of mild discomfort. In an environment of poverty, the disease's acute phase commonly lasts four to five days and usually entails a fever. Among poorly nourished children, report the authors of a WHO study, "a low-grade indisposition often continues for a month or more, sometimes as long as three months, with irregularly recurring loose stools, a progressively depleted nutritional state, and occasional recurrent acute episodes."[20] Some undernourished children suffer chronically recurring diarrhea for years.

In poor regions, one to four of every hundred children under the age of two who contracts diarrhea dies from it. In many parts of Latin America, the PAHO studies reveal, diarrhea caused a third or more of all deaths among those under five. In three Guatemalan villages studied in the 1950s, diarrhea accounted for 27 percent of all deaths in the *general* population, its toll especially great among small children. Yet, as surviving children gradually become acclimated to indigenous disease agents, their resistance increases. Then too, older children are for many reasons also more likely to be adequately fed. Thus, as children grow older, both the frequency with which they contract diarrhea and the affliction's death toll fall.

As this brief review implies, undernutrition's toll must be assessed in the total environment in which it occurs. Apart from diseases clearly linked to particular dietary deficiencies, undernutrition abets other disease agents surely and insidiously. Good health requires the elimination both of nutritional stress and of other environmental sources of illness— above all of unsanitary habitats. Even the most modern medical practices will be severely undermined when undernutrition is rampant.

Premature death is the cruelest sacrifice exacted by a social order that sanctions undernutrition. But other costs— also dreadful, if less absolute—may be borne by those surviving the combined ravages of poor diets and disease. Severe undernutrition in early childhood, growing evidence indicates, can stunt a child's physical and intellectual development. Combined with the social deprivations of poverty, undernutrition can impair reasoning powers, language and motor skills, and social behavior. If a child is underfed long enough during a critical period of development, no amount of compensatory feeding or education can fully restore what has been lost.

Although widely acknowledged by nutritionists and pediatricians, undernutrition's potential to inflict lasting personal damage may never be unequivocally established by usual scientific means and standards. The awesome complexities of the human mind, and of personality formation, assure uncertainty. While direct nutritional effects on the brain and nervous system are physical, the activity of thinking—however grounded in physical processes—involves impalpable acts of creation. To demonstrate an alteration in the number or size of certain brain cells is not necessarily to predict the resulting intellectual and behavioral consequences, and the classic enigmas of mind-body dualism remain as much the province of philosophy as of biology or chemistry.

The human brain does not mature by bread alone. Severe undernutrition virtually always occurs in a deprived social environment that can itself stunt intellectual development. Undernourished children are more apt than the well-fed to live in serious poverty, to suffer frequent illness, to have parents who are illiterate, and to be deprived of the enriching experiences that stimulate intellectual development. A lack of stimulation results in more than a gap in accumulated knowledge; it can, like nutritional deficiency, actually influence the brain's physical development.

Studies of humans and animals have proved that severe malnutrition early in life decreases the size of the brain and alters its cellular composition. What remains uncertain is the subsequent influence these changes exert on learning and behavior. Numerous studies of humans have clearly verified an association between severe early undernutrition and impaired learning abilities. While categorical claims of causation cannot be made, available evidence points strongly toward childhood undernutrition as one contributor to lifetime intellectual deficiencies. Following an exhaustive review of the research literature, a committee of the U.S. National Academy of Sciences has concluded that "the weight of evidence seems to indicate that early and severe malnutrition is an important factor in later intellectual development, above and beyond the effects of social-familial influences."[21]

An elaborate study in a Mexican village, for example, established that children who had recovered from severe undernutrition lagged behind others in developing both language skills and the ability to form concepts. Comparisons of stimulation in the home environment failed to explain the differences fully. Another study in Chile compared the intellectual performances of children malnourished in infancy to those of children who had been well-fed. While the two groups came from environments that were apparently almost identical in other respects, the formerly malnourished scored notably lower than their well-fed counterparts on intelligence tests.[22]

In 1964, researchers in Indonesia tested some children between the ages of five and twelve whose nutritional status in the late 1950s had been recorded in another study. All the 117 children studied came from the same low socioeconomic class. The investigators discovered that the children's intellectual as well as physical development could be predicted fairly accurately on the basis of their nutritional status during the preschool years. Previously malnourished children who had shown clinical signs of vitamin A deficiency between the ages of two and four scored lowest on intelligence tests, while those who had never been diagnosed as malnourished scored highest.[23]

The likelihood that such learning disabilities are in some measure irreversible emerges forbodingly from findings on the timing and nature of brain development. Like the rest of the body, the brain and its critical message systems do not grow uniformly throughout life; instead, most maturation takes place during a period of rapid development called the growth spurt. But the brain's growth spurt is far shorter than that of the rest of the body. At birth the human brain has already reached 25 percent of its adult weight, and after one year it weighs 70 percent of its adult potential. In contrast, overall body weight at birth is usually about 5 percent of that at maturity, and even at age ten, most people weigh only about half their adult total.

A particularly crucial attribute of the brain's growth spurt, which probably lasts from about the twentieth week of fetal life to two years after birth, is its apparent chronological inflexibility. The body seems to obey some inviolable time regulations; if certain kinds of growth do not occur within the specified period, the opportunity for that growth may be lost forever.[24] The period presents a once-in-a-lifetime opportunity for normal development, which is why undernutrition among pregnant women and small children has implications profoundly graver than those of undernutrition among any other group.

Fortunately, because human intellectual development is so wondrously complex, generalizations about the impact of nutritional deficiencies even in the initial years of life call for qualification. A recent study of Korean children who were adopted by U.S. parents underscores the potential of an exceptionally supportive social environment to mitigate the intellectual legacy of undernutrition. Those Korean-American school children who had exhibited signs of malnutrition when adopted (at an average age of eighteen months) now score as well on intelligence tests and perform as well in the classroom as the average U.S. child. On the other hand, those adopted Korean children who were well-fed in infancy score and perform *better* than the average child in the United States. Thus, the formerly malnourished still lag behind those with comparable home environments.[25]

Virtually all research on the intellectual impact of dietary deficiencies has focused on people suffering from severe protein-calorie malnutrition. Children once hospitalized with identifiable acute conditions such as marasmus or kwashiorkor are most often studied. But for every child who is severely undernourished, many more suffer milder chronic dietary deficiencies. To determine whether moderate undernutrition can also wreak lasting intellectual damage is to describe the fate of untold numbers of children.

Clearly, moderate undernutrition and a colorless social environment together impair a child's later intellectual performance, but their relative importance has not been ascertained. The U. S. National Academy of Sciences has declared that studies relating "moderate malnutrition . . . to later intellectual performance have frequently found that malnutrition does play a role apart from factors related to social status. This is a tentative conclusion, however, and confirmation awaits more systematic research." Studies of animal brain development support this position; some tests have revealed that the cerebral cortexes develop incompletely in animals suffering even moderate undernutrition throughout critical periods in early life.[26]

The debate over the exact roles of early undernutrition and social deprivation in impairing learning abilities is academic. The two negative forces virtually always coexist, reinforcing each other. Moreover, apart from inflicting possible harm upon the brain and nervous system, undernutrition can impair intellectual development by indirectly affecting personality formation. Undernutrition accentuates—and even creates—the paucity of stimulation and experience that hinders personal development. Often apathetic and socially withdrawn, the poorly nourished tend to be less sociable than the well-fed. Physical and mental fatigue, the inability to concentrate, and low motivation all doom them to poor performance at school; and frequent illness means frequent absence from the classroom. Poorly nourished children thus fall behind in a critical learning period, suffering what Alan Berg has called "an irreversible loss of opportunity," whether or not their brains have been physically damaged.[27]

Perhaps the chief lesson of the still incomplete research record on nutrition and learning is that undernutrition, disease, and poverty are deeply interwoven. Good nutrition alone will not ward off poverty nor erase its scars, but even the most creative educational efforts may fail in the face of undernutrition. Our knowledge of human brain development imparts a special urgency to efforts to provide an adequate diet to pregnant and nursing mothers and to children under two years old. At the same time, ample evidence shows that improved diets and social conditions at any stage of life benefit the individual.

Throughout history, many forces have influenced food-consumption patterns, but health considerations have not always been among them. Long lacking both the medical knowledge and the agricultural resources needed to promote healthy diets, humanity now has both, and governments seriously committed to the project can now reduce malnutrition markedly. Nutrition strategies, with which governments influence people's diets, are increasingly recognized as a public responsibility. In a growing number of poor countries, the idea of national planning for improved nutrition has already caught on—though much remains to be done.

Observing the strong correlation between poverty and nutrition, some analysts view adopting nutrition strategies as an unnecessary diversion from the overriding task of raising the incomes of the poor. According to various versions of this perspective, hastening economic growth, redistributing income, or both are the best defenses against undernutrition. While based on truths, such arguments can be dangerously incomplete. Setting minimum income levels is certainly a necessary part of any strategy for stamping out undernutrition, but it is seldom all that is needed. While the poor must have land, jobs, and decent incomes if undernutrition is to be obliterated, the positive impact of all three on diets can be enhanced when combined with careful attention to the nutrition factor.

At the rates of economic growth foreseeable in many poor countries, decades or even centuries will pass before the threat of undernutrition fades away. In fact, if the economic growth patterns now prevailing in many countries persist, the landless, the small-scale farmers, and the urban slum dwellers, among others, may derive little benefit from increases in the gross national product—even when these increases reflect gains in agricultural production. The GNP is simply not an adequate gauge of progress in meeting human needs.

For example, Brazilian farmers have taken advantage of the tight world protein market by rapidly increasing their production of soybeans, most of which they sell abroad for livestock feed. But to do so, farmers have planted soybeans on land formerly used to grow the traditional bean crop—the staple protein food eaten by low-income families. Partly because of this diversion of farmlands, per capita production of food beans in Brazil fell by one-third between 1971 and 1974, and their price tripled. In effect, rich European and Japanese consumers bid protein away from Brazil's poor. The Brazilian GNP received a healthy boost, national foreign-exchange reserves were bolstered, and soybean farmers prospered—but undernutrition undoubtedly grew more severe among Brazil's poor.

One way countries can help assure that nutritional considerations receive high priority is to establish a government agency to monitor nutrition trends and to weigh the nutritional implications of major policies and programs. Using analyses of the nutritional impacts of various institutions and projects, governments could decide to avoid, alter, or offset those development paths, such as Brazil's recent soybean boom, that entail negative health repercussions. At the least, those in power would be forced to confront openly the human consequences of the programs they engineer. Furthermore, systematic nutritional scanning can help draw attention to the changes needed to improve diets—whether land reforms, food supplements, or job creation. Documenting hardship and inequity can itself right no wrongs, but it is a critical preamble to action. In the United States, for example, the shocking findings of nutritional surveys in the late 1960s prompted the government to expand substantially its food-assistance programs for the poor.

Nutrition planning cannot substitute for economic growth, but setting nutritional priorities can help give growth a human face. Nor is a nutrition strategy a surrogate for fundamental reforms in the distribution of land and income. But a strategy can, perhaps, spur the redistribution of productive resources. Where growing populations overwhelm the local environment and food-production capacity, nutrition planning cannot compensate for a dangerously high birth rate. But it can prompt policymakers to accord higher priority to the family-planning services, education, medical care, and improved diets that promote the norm of the small family.

Beyond the sway that nutrition planning can exert on the broad directions of national development, it can lead to the adoption of more specific nutritional programs that have already proven effective in various countries. Just as fortifying bread, milk, and salt wiped out many vitamin-deficiency diseases in the West, for instance, adding nutrients to various foods is paying off in many poor countries today. Adding iodine to salt has greatly reduced goiter in Guatemala, and fortifying buns with protein is cutting undernutrition among school children in the Philippines. But fortification's potential is far from fully realized. Special efforts to provide direct food supplements to needy infants and to pregnant and nursing mothers may have even greater benefits, especially in view of the evidence that lasting damage to a person's learning ability and health can result from undernutrition early in life.

Nutrition education—for doctors and other adults as well as for children—can in principle improve the health of people at any income level. According to WHO estimates, one-half or more of the nutritional problems of Africa could be solved by education. There and elsewhere, ignorance about the nutritional value of local foods, misconceptions about the appropriateness of certain diets for infants and pregnant women, and traditional food-allocation patterns within the family all foster undernutrition.[28]

Campaigns to halt the disastrous decline in breast feeding are needed throughout Africa, Asia, and Latin America—where the economic and sanitary prerequisites of a healthful transition to bottle feeding still do not exist and where high-quality protein is usually scarce. In his comprehensive review of the role of nutrition in development, Alan Berg concludes that efforts to halt the abandonment of breast feeding "may be of greater significance than any other form of nutrition intervention."[29] Lactation not only provides nutritious, sanitary food to the infant, but also often has a contraceptive effect on the mother by delaying the onset of ovulation after pregnancy. Hence, investments in health care, nutrition programs, agricultural development, and family planning are all undercut to some degree when lactation is cut back.

Developing countries bent upon preserving the practice of breast feeding and upon preventing the ravages of misused bottle feeding must move on two fronts. They must undertake mass education programs, and they must control strictly the advertising and sales practices of infant-formula sellers. Prospective mothers and their families need to understand both the marked health advantages to the child of breast feeding and the nursing mother's need for extra food. Effective education must somehow set right the bogus association—encouraged by irresponsible advertising—of expensive canned preparations with vigorous and contented babies. More specifically, governments and health workers must spread word of the tremendous health benefits of nursing in the initial half year of life, the insidious impact of bottle feeding under prevailing social conditions, and (especially in the poorest regions) the nutritional advantages of continuing to nurse children into their second year of life. Educational programs are often needed for doctors, too, who sometimes cooperate with infant-food companies or otherwise discourage nursing.

The subjects of extensive public scrutiny in recent years, many of the large international manufacturers of infant formulas and foods have pledged to self-regulate more scrupulously their marketing techniques in poor countries. Still, governmental regulation of sales and sales methods remains a prime need. Local distributors or manufacturers may utterly disregard the pledges issued at the faraway headquarters of the multinational companies—and even the pledged changes in marketing practices may be inadequate. Some mothers simply cannot breast feed, and inexpensive, nutritious supplemental foods can—if properly used—contribute to a child's development after the early months. However, shaping the role for infant-food manufacturers needs to be the province of public policy rather than that of the private market.

Getting working mothers to breast-feed presents an especially tenacious problem, one that will grow as more and more women find social roles outside the home. A possible partial solution is to establish nurseries in workplaces and to schedule special nursing breaks during the day. Just such a program has helped maintain breast feeding in the Soviet Union on a wide scale. In the factories of the developing world, social accounting of the total costs of *not* nursing will help justify such additional expenses.

Widespread appreciation of the significance of the breast-to-bottle transition must precede effective national action to protect infant health and nutrition. Cornell University physician Michael C. Latham writes that "in several developing countries where I have worked, bottle feeding is the cause of more deaths than is cancer—yet vast sums are spent on cancer research, journals and textbooks are devoted to tumors, while research on breast feeding is quite limited and the literature on the subject is rather scanty."[30] Fortunately, the recent flurry of pronouncements from international organizations and in medical writings on infant-feeding practices suggests that breast feeding may at last begin receiving the priority attention it deserves. If what is obviously a deeply rooted social trend can be turned around, millions of lives will be saved and millions more will be bettered.

4. Mutinous Bounty: Hazards of the Affluent Diet*

THE STAMP of each culture's cuisine is unique; Americans have hamburgers, the French rich sauces, the Japanese raw fish. Nevertheless, the basic nutritional components, if not the particular dishes, of all diets invite comparisons. And such comparisons reveal that over the last century or so a consumption pattern sometimes called the "affluent diet" has taken hold in the industrial Western countries.

The affluent diet flourishes only where incomes range far above subsistence level and where people have market access to the bounty of a highly productive agricultural system —hence its name. Those with an affluent diet consume large amounts of animal proteins and fats as meats and dairy products; they substitute highly refined flour and sugar for bulky carbohydrates like whole grains, tubers, fruits, and vegetables; and, increasingly, they choose commercially manufactured foods over unprocessed products.

The affluent diet is most deeply entrenched in North America, but it has taken hold in Western Europe too. Japan and the Soviet Union, slower to abandon traditional grain or potato-centered diets, are quickly making up for lost time.

---

* I appreciate Frank Record's help in preparing this chapter.

The "refined" meat-heavy diet is also enticing the urban elite in Africa, Asia, and Latin America. At the marketplace and at the dinner table, the appeals of meat, refined flour, and sugar are proving stronger than dietary traditions. Never before this century have so many eaten so "well."

But is eating the affluent diet eating well? By traditional nutritional measures, the answer would seem to be yes. The affluent diet supplies protein in generous amounts, energy in adequate—even excessive—amounts, and key vitamins and minerals. It is also a good defense against age-old nutrient-deficiency diseases such as scurvy and pellagra.

Nutritional appearances, however, can deceive. Observed links between the way people in the industrial countries eat and the way they live and die have cast the soundness of the affluent diet into doubt. Such connections have forced nutritionists and doctors to consider this diet from new angles, and to refigure the meaning of "good nutrition." They have also forced experts to evaluate a diet within the context of a particular lifestyle. Sobering conclusions emerge from this reassessment: like most get-rich-quick schemes, the quest for rich foods entails grave risks.

The most suspect characteristics of the affluent diet are its high levels of fats, especially animal fats, and cholesterol. As most people know, greasy fried foods, butter, and salad oil contain fats; but fewer realize that much of the fat we eat comes in subtler forms. Meats, especially beef and pork (which contain more fat than do poultry and fish), and dairy products also add fat to the diet. Cholesterol, known for its association with circulatory ailments, is most concentrated in eggs and liver; but other animal products also contain cholesterol.

Among Westerners, fats have accounted for an increasing proportion of total caloric intake over the last century. Largely because they eat more meat and dairy products, people in the industrial countries consume far more fat than those, such as the Greeks, with oilier-looking cuisines. Fats sometimes account for 45 to 50 percent of the calories in a North American's diet. The national average is over 40 percent in the United States and in many Western countries, while fats comprise less than a fourth of the food energy consumed by those in most poor countries.

The kind, as well as the quantity, of fat that people eat has health implications. A high intake of saturated fats, supplied mainly by animal products, may promote cardiovascular problems and, possibly, some cancers. Unsaturated fats seem to entail fewer health risks, but they still appear dangerous when consumed at high levels.

Opposing forces have influenced the consumption of vegetable and animal fats in developed countries. Financial and health considerations have prompted people to switch from butter to vegetable-based margarines and from lard to hydrogenated vegetable oils. At the same time, climbing meat consumption has partially offset these health benefits. Overall, animal-fat intake remains high and total fat consumption has been driven upward.

Average consumption of meats and poultry in the United States, Australia, and Argentina has now leveled off at close to 250 pounds (carcass weight) a year per capita. In France, West Germany, and Canada, consumption now amounts to 200 pounds per person a year, while other Europeans eat smaller but generally increasing amounts of meat. The Japanese lag conspicuously behind those in other rich countries in meat consumption, but Japan's per capita intake of forty-four pounds in 1974 represented a spectacular 428 percent jump over the 1961 level. In contrast, the average person in many poor countries eats fewer than twenty pounds of meat a year.

Although *total* grain use in the developed countries has risen markedly over recent decades, the fat-rich affluent diet is low in whole grains. Ranging up to 1600 pounds per capita, grain consumption now averages two to five times that in poorer countries; but a large share of the total is consumed indirectly as meat from grain-fed animals. Thus the possible benefits of whole grains are forfeited to animals even as we enrich our diets with fat. The popularity of "prime" beef, the highly marbled type for which consumers pay premium prices, exemplifies this changeover perfectly. Prime beef is the flesh of cattle raised partly on feedlots where about ten pounds of grain are consumed for every pound of meat added during the stay. Since grain-fed beef contains more fat than range-fed beef does, people pay extra for a product that, at current consumption levels in many countries, is more likely than less fatty meats to threaten their well-being.

Even the grain that remains in the affluent diet is stripped of most of the fiber, or roughage. Wheat is usually milled into refined white flour. Raw or lightly cooked fruits and vegetables, which also provide fiber, are increasingly being passed over in favor of canned or frozen foods, which are often overcooked. Those fruits and vegetables that are bought fresh are often peeled or overcooked before they are eaten. Reducing dietary fiber in this manner apparently alters the chemistry of digestion, in turn possibly promoting various diseases of the digestive system.

Starch intake has dropped precipitously along with the consumption of bulky foods and fiber in the affluent diet, and sugar intake is rising. While few traditional societies use refined sugar at all, and recipes calling for sugar were rare in Europe and North America a century back, high sugar consumption now plagues all the developed and many less developed countries. Globally, per capita sugar consumption has grown by half just since 1950, and the average person in the world now eats forty-four pounds of sugar a year. Cubans, Costa Ricans, Americans, Australians, and Israelis each down over a hundred pounds of sugar a year, while Western Europeans eat an average of ninety pounds each. In contrast, annual sugar consumption in Japan, Taiwan, and the Philippines, though climbing fast, is about fifty pounds per person; and sugar intake in many poor countries is much lower still. As the world's sweet tooth grows, so do its dental bills. An obvious contributor to tooth decay, high sugar consumption may—some researchers contend—also be linked to obesity, diabetes, and other diseases.

As the affluent diet has spread, so have many once rare diseases such as coronary heart disease, diabetes, diverticulosis, and bowel cancer. Confined primarily to those leading the lifestyles of the developed Western world, whether in Paris or Singapore, these ailments have been appropriately tagged the "diseases of civilization." Where they prevail, improved sanitation and ample food supplies have largely stamped out fatal infections and undernutrition—which have been replaced by modern diseases that strike not only the old. Some ingredients of modern Western life—and dietary factors are among the leading suspects—are abetting these killers.

Medical detectives are slowly unraveling the tangled interconnections that link the affluent diet to the various diseases of civilization. Combined with a sedentary lifestyle, high calorie consumption leads to obesity, which in turn encourages diabetes, hypertension, and coronary heart disease. High intake of refined foods such as white flour and sugar may encourage diverticulosis and other conditions, while high salt intake possibly promotes hypertension. (Diabetes and hypertension, sometimes directly lethal, greatly boost the risk of coronary heart disease and, for those suffering from hypertension, stroke.) A diet high in animal fats fosters arterial problems that can lead to a coronary attack or stroke. Finally, excessive dietary fats may also be linked to the genesis of bowel, breast, prostate, and other types of cancer.

Both affluent diets and sedentary lifestyles represent radical departures from the conditions under which humans evolved for millions of years. That our bodies rebel should scarcely surprise us.

Human beings long depended upon their legs for transportation and upon their physical strength for the cultivation of food. The overwhelming majority consumed just enough to survive while the privileged few wore obesity like a status symbol. Indeed, the Roman senator's girth won him great prestige among the mass of underfed plebeians, and Aga Khan's yearly weighings were legendary among his people. Today the same attitudes still prevail in many less developed countries.

In North America, Europe, and other developed areas, most people from all social classes now get more than enough to eat, and obesity is no longer the "privilege" of the elite. In fact, excessive fat has become the scourge of the lower class and, to the many Westerners who prize leanness, a mark of social disdain. "Doppelkinnepidemie," the double-chin epidemic, has blossomed in West Germany since the postwar economic miracle. In the United States, 10 to 20 percent of all children and 35 to 50 percent of the middle-aged are overweight.

The increased prevalence of obesity is not, however, solely a function of changing food supplies and of mercurial attitudes about the ideal weight. Combined with individual genetic susceptibility to obesity, two factors—caloric intake and the expenditure of energy through physical activity— determine weight gains. In some rich countries calorie consumption has actually fallen since the turn of the century, but not as rapidly as the rate at which people's exercise has declined.[1] In the age of machine labor, fewer and fewer jobs require physical work of any sort. Even the modern farmer, perched atop his tractor, can be overweight and out of condition. Millions of office workers get no exercise whatever, save a short walk or an occasional sprint to catch the rush-hour bus. In today's sedentary civilizations, the new species of *Homo sedentarius* has migrated from the cities and the suburbs to the countryside.

Obesity, often defined as the condition of being 20 percent or more over a desirable weight determined mainly on the basis of mortality statistics, is not randomly distributed throughout society. Rather, in developed countries, the condition seems to be concentrated in the lowest socioeconomic groups. A study performed in New York City showed that one of every three lower-class women is obese, compared to one in twenty among upper-class women. Similarly, obesity is more common among lower-class six-year-olds than among their upper-class counterparts.[2]

More than a social problem, obesity interests the medical profession because obese people run a higher risk of premature death than other people do. For example, men who are 10 percent overweight have a one-third higher mortality rate in any given year than those of average weight, primarily because of their exceptional susceptibility to high blood pressure, diabetes, and coronary heart disease. Death rates among men more than 20 percent overweight are elevated by 50 percent. According to leading U.S. health officials, an estimated one-fifth of all Americans are so overweight that their health is threatened.[3] Hippocrates' dictum that the fat die sooner than the thin rings as true today as it did two thousand years ago.

Fortunately, obesity and its ill effects can often be totally reversed. Diabetes and hypertension often disappear along with excess weight. Data from life insurance companies show that when obese people lose and keep off weight, their life expectancy rises to what it would have been had they never been obese. However, overfeeding early in life may, some researchers believe, produce extra fat cells that then contribute to obesity for the rest of a person's life. At least four out of five obese children become obese adults. (One factor that many nutritionists link to a higher incidence of obesity among children is the substitution of bottle feeding for breast feeding; mothers who force their babies to finish their bottles may be encouraging more than baby fat.)[4]

Some obese children habitually eat too much, but studies have shown that low physical activity often figures centrally in their weight gains as well. Many overweight children do not eat much more than their classmates do, but they are more apt to be inactive.[5] Yet why both obese children and obese adults are so inactive remains a medical mystery.

Crash diets undertaken at any age, however effective in the short term, are rarely beneficial over time unless followed by increased routine physical activity and by a permanent reduction in caloric intake. For many, a daily caloric excess equivalent to half a slice of bread or half a glass of beer can result in a weight gain of more than forty pounds within ten years. A reduction in daily exercise by the equivalent of a ten-minute walk can have the same effect.[6]

Enamored of mechanical convenience and conveyance, many people engage in so little physical activity that simply eating to the point of feeling satisfied means eating excess calories. Studies show that, in the words of nutritionist Jean Mayer, "decreasing activity below a certain limit will no longer be accompanied by a decrease in appetite."[7] Thus both sides of the diet-exercise equation must be considered if life-threatening fat is to be trimmed.

Seldom has one disease dominated an era as coronary heart disease dominates our own. Once a rare affliction even among the aged, it is now the leading killer of the old and the middle-aged in many countries; and it sometimes takes the lives of the young as well. The affluent diet and sedentary lifestyles are contributing to this trend in both the developed world and in the cities of the poor countries.

All cardiovascular diseases together, including coronary

heart disease, strokes, arterial diseases, and others, account
for about *one half* of all deaths in the industrialized countries. Coronary heart disease, which involves the coronary
arteries through which the heart supplies itself with blood,
often culminates in a "heart attack" when the blood supply
is blocked. This disease accounts for one in every three
deaths in many developed countries, including the United
States, where it claims some 700,000 lives each year. In Japan
and France, cerebrovascular disease, or stroke, which involves an impaired supply of blood to parts of the brain, takes
even more lives than does coronary heart disease.

World Health Organization data for eighteen Western
countries reveal increases in the incidence of coronary heart
disease between 1950 and 1968 for every age group. Among
those aged thirty-five to forty-four, the incidence rose by
more than 50 percent; and, among those aged forty-five to
fifty-four, by more than 30 percent. In the United States,
where coronary fatalities are more prevalent than in any
other large country, the frequency of deaths from this disease for most age groups has tapered off somewhat since the
early 1960s. Improved medical treatment of heart-disease
victims and changing lifestyles have probably contributed to
this downturn. In the United Kingdom, too, the coronary
death rate among men has stopped rising since 1965. But
incidence rates are climbing throughout most of the world.[8]

In India, what sketchy information exists shows that the
number of coronary patients in urban hospitals has been
increasing steadily over the past twenty years. The incidence
of heart attacks is on the rise in China, Sri Lanka, Korea,
Malaysia, and the Philippines too. In seventeen out of
twenty-two countries in North and South America, the disease is now one of the five principal causes of death. In ten
of these countries, heart disease is the number one killer.[9]

Although it has tripled over the last fifteen years, Japan's
coronary death rate is still low compared to that in other

developed countries, quite possibly because the Japanese consume relatively little animal fat. Yet high saturated-fat consumption is only one of the "risk factors" that have been associated with heart attacks. Others include obesity, high blood cholesterol, diabetes, hypertension, sedentary living, stress, and cigarette smoking. Higher-than-normal risks are also run by males, heavy drinkers, those with a family history of the disease, and those who drink soft (mineral-free) water.

Doctors use the term "risk factor" rather than the term "cause" to discuss the traits associated with an increased propensity to developing heart disease. They do so in part because few cause-and-effect relationships have been absolutely established in this area of inquiry, and in part because no single "cause" can usually be held accountable for the present epidemic of degenerative diseases.

The contribution of various risk-factors to heart-attack odds has been the subject of the noted Framingham study. Since 1948, doctors have examined more than five thousand men and women in Framingham, Massachusetts, for the initial development of coronary disease. Angina pectoris, or chest pain, which is frequently an early indicator of coronary disease, is more common among obese men both with and without elevated blood pressure and blood cholesterol. Yet for women, obesity does not increase the chances of angina unless accompanied by high blood pressure and high levels of blood cholesterol.

Risk factors associated with heart disease combine in deadly patterns. A forty-five-year-old American man who smokes more than a pack of cigarettes a day doubles his chances of a heart attack. But the forty-five-year-old smoker with high blood pressure and a high blood-cholesterol level runs nearly *four times* the risk of a heart attack than does a nonsmoker with normal blood-pressure and cholesterol levels.[10]

Socioeconomic levels also correlate with the incidence of

coronary disease in the United States. As median family incomes rise, coronary death rates drop. The upper-middle and middle classes in the United States suffer from proportionately less coronary disease than they did before World War II, and both have lower coronary death rates than the poor. Apparently, the rich in the United States are now more aware than the poor of the various risk factors associated with heart attacks, and some have changed their ways accordingly. But those in the lower economic classes have rushed to embrace the same affluent diets and sedentary lifestyles that only the wealthy once claimed. Whether the U.S. pattern of rising and falling heart-disease rates will typify development in other countries is an open question. Many premature coronary deaths in developing countries could probably be avoided, however, if public health authorities would establish programs to help people skirt known risks.

In ways but poorly understood, hereditary factors also influence the development of coronary heart disease. In Finland, the difference in coronary mortality rates between the eastern and western parts of the country is apparently partly genetic in origin. Genetically predisposed to the early onset of atherosclerosis (*and* raised on a diet extremely high in animal fats), adults from the East have the world's highest recorded coronary death rate.[11] But some individuals in every country are predisposed to developing coronary disease.

Women seem to be partially protected from atherosclerosis and heart attacks by female sex hormones. During the twelve-year Framingham study, 252 men and only 128 women developed coronary heart disease. Moreover, the stricken men developed much more serious forms of the disease than did the women. Female coronary disease rates are affected by lifestyle and diet, just as male rates are, but the gap in coronary disease incidence between the sexes is nevertheless large.[12]

Atherosclerosis, the accumulation of fatty deposits and tissue in the arteries, seems to be influenced by the consumption of saturated fats and cholesterol. These food components appear to help trigger the chain of events that leads from a high cholesterol blood count first to atherosclerosis and then to a completely blocked coronary artery and a heart attack.

Just what determines cholesterol levels in the blood and how a high blood-cholesterol level promotes atherosclerosis are as yet unknown. But considerable evidence shows that a diet high in unsaturated fats lowers the body's output of cholesterol, while a high intake of saturated fats apparently stimulates the liver to produce more cholesterol. Cholesterol levels in the bloodstream may also be raised by high consumption of cholesterol-rich foods. Other factors—weight, exercise, and heredity among them—seem to affect the body's cholesterol production as well. According to the U.S. National Academy of Sciences and the American Medical Association, there is "abundant evidence that the risk of developing coronary heart disease is positively correlated with the level of cholesterol in the (blood) plasma . . . and that the level of cholesterol can be lowered by appropriate dietary modifications."[13]

Coronary heart disease was christened the "doctors' disease" when the association between the stressful lives of doctors and their relatively high susceptibility to heart attacks was first noticed in the nineteenth century. Some researchers today also contend that coronary disease and competitive, stressful living go hand in hand. The body reacts to mental stress by releasing into the bloodstream various hormones that affect the way the body breaks down fats and cholesterol. Yet diet can apparently alter the effects of stress on blood cholesterol. As one heart specialist hypothesizes, "The potential for harm to the cardiovascular system by stressful patterns of living is markedly diminished if not nullified by subsistence on a diet low in fat."[14]

While researchers have yet to prove that exercise retards or stops arterial clogging, many authorities believe that it can and that regular exercise reduces both a person's likelihood of contracting coronary heart disease and the damage such disease can do. Regular exercise in conjunction with a controlled-fat diet, a recent U.S. study showed, help to reduce blood cholesterol and to maintain it at a low level. Regular exercise also increases the supply of oxygen to the muscles and makes the heart work more economically, and may thus help defend a person against heart attack.[15]

Medical authorities in the United States, Sweden, Norway, the United Kingdom, and elsewhere all exhort adults to reduce fat consumption. In their view, fats should supply less than 35 percent of total calories, as opposed to the 40–45 percent now common in these countries. Furthermore, according to the American Heart Association and others, most adult males should sharply reduce their daily cholesterol intake to no more than 300 milligrams.[16] (One egg contains 250 mgs. of cholesterol, while a three-ounce cooked piece of beef, pork, or chicken contains approximately eighty-five mgs.)

No diet and no amount of exercise can eliminate coronary heart disease. Elderly people, as well as younger people genetically predisposed to the disease, will continue to succumb to heart attacks. However, hundreds of thousands of deaths each year from coronary disease could probably be prevented and could certainly be postponed if changes in diet and lifestyle were made. In the rich countries, signs of atherosclerosis now appear in teenagers as well as in the middle-aged. About 45 percent of all young American men have significant atherosclerosis by age twenty-five.[17] Thus, measures aimed at preventing heart disease must be introduced early in life and must be long-lasting.

Hypertension, or high blood pressure, is now one of the most common illnesses in the world. The prevalence of hypertension in affluent nations is widely recognized; the emergence of this disease in the cities of the world's poorer countries is less so. Salt intake, genetic factors, stress, and urbanization all seem to be associated with rises in the incidence of hypertension in New York's boroughs and in São Paulo's *favelas*.

High blood pressure goes undetected in many people. But the ailments it promotes—coronary heart disease, stroke, congestive heart failure, kidney disease, and others—are all too obvious when they strike. The extensive Framingham heart study showed that two out of every three middle-aged people with a history of stroke or coronary heart disease had above-normal blood pressure.

Hypertension can shorten its victims' lives. A thirty-five-year-old American man with blood pressure 14 percent above normal for his age has lost about nine years of his life expectancy. A forty-five-year-old man whose blood pressure is 17 percent or more above normal is running twice the risk of a heart attack and four times the risk of a stroke that a man with blood pressure slightly lower than normal faces.[18]

In nearly all cases the actual cause of hypertension is unknown. But dietary factors, especially salt intake levels, are now the subject of many medical studies. Past research has firmly established the link between high salt consumption and high blood pressure in rats. While only circumstantial, the evidence strongly suggests that high salt intake contributes significantly to hypertension in humans too.

The late Dr. Lewis K. Dahl, who studied hypertension in rats as well as in human beings, found that a low-salt diet drove down blood pressure levels not only for hypertensives in general, but also for obese people in particular. Obesity has been clearly established as a risk factor for both coronary heart disease and hypertension, and obese people who adopt special low-salt, low-calorie diets reduce their blood pressure readings long before they lose weight. Studies of people in the Bahamas, South Africa, Japan, and Polynesia have all shown associations between high salt intake and high blood pressure.[19]

The average person in an industrial country consumes at least ten times more salt than the body actually requires.[20] However, some individuals consume large amounts of salt without ever developing hypertension. Dahl and others postulated and determined experimentally in rats that genetic predisposition plays a key role in this process. Thus, some individuals may be so predisposed to hypertension that small amounts of salt can produce the disease. At the other extreme, those who are not so predisposed may be able to eat as much salt as they please without fear of consequences.

The hypertension rates of cultural subgroups within countries and among different countries vary with salt consumption levels. "Without exception, low blood pressure societies are low salt societies," says Dr. Lot B. Page of Tufts University. In Japan, where northerners eat more salt than do southerners, the greater incidence of hypertension in the North is apparently salt-related. On average, Japanese have perhaps the world's highest salt consumption rate, which may help explain their exceptional susceptibility to hypertension and strokes.[21]

Some doctors believe that a difference in salt consumption rates helps explain why proportionately more U.S. blacks than U.S. whites suffer from hypertension, but the dietary surveys needed to prove such a relationship have not been carried out. Twenty-two percent of blacks, compared to 15 percent of the white population, have dangerously elevated blood pressure. Other researchers explain the high incidence of hypertension among blacks as a consequence of life in urban ghettos and of the abnormal stresses associated with social and economic discrimination. Many feel that stress and high salt intake work together insidiously to promote hypertension.[22]

Work-related tedium or stress, as well as certain minerals

found in some drinking water, can apparently promote abnormally high blood pressure.[23] Family background also seems to affect individual susceptibility to hypertension: a child with a hypertensive parent is more apt to develop the disease than a child from a family free of hypertension. Also, for unknown reasons, older children in large families tend to have higher blood pressure than their younger sisters and brothers.

Although uncertainties shroud its cause, hypertension can often be controlled with modern drugs. Yet, even people genetically predisposed to hypertension might completely avoid the disease by minding their diets.

As the affluent diet has spread, the incidence of diabetes has risen apace. In poor countries, diabetes appears to be mainly an urban disease; in rich countries, it afflicts urban and rural residents alike.

In the United States in 1900, diabetes was the twenty-seventh most common cause of death. By the mid-1970s, it had captured fifth place. According to the National Commission on Diabetes, the number of reported cases in the United States jumped 50 percent from 1965 to 1973. If the heart diseases, circulatory problems, kidney disorders, and other potentially fatal complications of diabetes are added to its annual direct death toll, diabetes emerges as the third most important killer, trailing only cardiovascular disease and cancer. In the United States, the United Kingdom, and elsewhere, the disease is also a major cause of blindness.[24]

A rich urban resident in India, surveys show, is about twice as likely as his poor rural countryman to develop diabetes. A similar trend among those people who have only recently been exposed to the affluent lifestyle of the capital city was discovered by a medical researcher in Dakar, Senegal. The number of diabetics in Dakar's clinics increased from twenty-one to 963 between the years 1965 and 1970.[25]

Many people think of diabetes as a childhood disease that

has been brought under control through the use of insulin. In fact, insulin has prolonged the life of juvenile diabetics, but its ready availability has not prevented a tremendous increase in the number of middle-aged or elderly victims of what is called the "maturity-onset" variety of the disease. Juvenile diabetics usually have such low levels of insulin that they could not live without regular injections of this hormone. But maturity-onset diabetics often have only slight deficiencies, and their insulin levels are influenced highly by the amount and type of food they eat.

In many countries the incidence of the late-blooming type of diabetes is about four times higher than that of the juvenile type, and the margin is widening. The number of maturity-onset victims in Japan in the last two decades of rapid economic growth has increased noticeably, but cases of juvenile diabetes among Japanese under forty are no more frequent than they were twenty years ago. Diabetes was extremely rare among middle-aged Japanese females at the end of World War II, but had become the eighth leading cause of death among this age group by 1972.[26]

Obesity fosters diabetes in those genetically predisposed to the disease. Dr. George Cahill, Chief of the Joslin Diabetes Research Center in Boston, recently stressed the catalytic role of overeating, saying: "Overnutrition unmasks the diabetic. The greatest portion of diabetes we have here in this country is frankly due just to overnutrition." Some researchers also suspect that diabetes can be promoted by a sugar-laden diet. Since a person who is 20 percent overweight is more than twice as likely as a person of normal weight to develop diabetes, moderation at the table and regular exercise may help prevent this unwanted offspring of the affluent diet among those genetically susceptible to the disease.[27]

Connections between the affluent diet and cardiovascular diseases have long been postulated by many doctors. Today the medical case against this diet is broadening as a result of research into the origins of cancer. Some of the major lethal cancers in Europe and North America, including malignancies of the colon, rectum, breast, and prostate gland, appear to be linked to the affluent diet. However, the exact nature of those links is unproven, as the current debate over bowel cancer illustrates. (Numerous other suspected dietary influences on cancer are discussed in Chapter 5.)

Although rare elsewhere, bowel cancer is one of the most common malignancies found in the developed Western nations. In the United Kingdom and the United States, it is second only to lung cancer as a source of cancer deaths. The striking international differences in incidence must stem from environmental rather than genetic factors: for example, Japanese who migrate to the United States succumb to bowel cancer at the high U.S. rates rather than at the low Japanese ones. Two theories on the causes of bowel cancer, one centered on dietary fiber and the other on dietary fat, have gained wide credence in recent years. Either or both may be correct to some degree, but neither has been firmly established.

Not yet precisely defined, fiber (or roughage) is usually thought of as the indigestible part of plant cell-walls. Fiber exists mainly in the outer layers of grain kernels and in raw or lightly cooked fruits and vegetables. It adds bulk to the diet and it also absorbs water and swells in the stomach and intestines. The stools of those with high-fiber diets are softer and larger than the stools often associated with the low-fiber diet, and they tend to pass through the body more quickly. The consumption-to-elimination process often lasts three or more days for Westerners, whose diet contains less fiber than it once did, while it averages only a day or two for traditional African villagers, whose diet is high in fiber and among whom bowel cancer is rare.

Bowel cancer is caused, many believe, by carcinogenic

substances produced by bacteria in the colon. A highly refined diet may alter the composition of the colonic bacteria, encouraging those species that are most likely to degrade digestive substances into carcinogens. Since the low-fiber stool remains in the bowel longer, natural intestinal bacteria have more time to create carcinogens in any case. Finally, the relatively dense low-fiber stool may expose the colon wall to higher concentrations of these carcinogens.[28]

Critics have pointed out several weaknesses in the fiber theory. That the actual concentration of carcinogens in the stool is higher with a refined diet has not been proven to the satisfaction of many. And a faster rate of stool passage through the colon does not necessarily mean that any particular point on the colon wall receives less exposure to carcinogens; the net effect of frequent short exposures could equal that of fewer, longer exposures. Most damaging of all to the theory are the results of the few available surveys comparing the diets and cancer rates of various populations.

While bowel cancer does indeed tend to be far more common in countries with affluent diets than in developing countries, a comparison of populations in thirty-seven countries revealed no statistically significant correlation between average fiber intake and colon-cancer rates. Similarly, a study of rising bowel-cancer rates among Japanese immigrants and their children in Hawaii failed to uncover a statistical correlation between dietary fiber intake and cancer trends.[29] The inadequate definition and measurement of fiber, and the resultant muddled state of international statistics on fiber consumption, may conceal a true connection. But until statistical comparisons reveal a meaningful association, the case for a causal relationship between fiber and cancer will remain weak.

The hypothesis that higher fat consumption rather than lower fiber consumption promotes bowel cancer rests upon somewhat firmer empirical foundations. Some scientists contend that high-fat foods change the composition of intestinal bacteria and promote the production of bile acids that are transformed into carcinogens within the colon.[30] The thirty-seven-country comparison just noted revealed that fat and animal-protein consumption levels correlated more clearly with colon-cancer rates than did any other variables measured.

Breast cancer appears internationally in almost exactly the same pattern as bowel cancer. It strikes more women in the United States and Western Europe than does any other malignancy, yet it is comparatively rare throughout the developing world. While Japanese women seldom develop breast tumors, their chances of doing so begin to rise when they move to the United States and adopt a new way of life.

The close international correlation of bowel-cancer and breast-cancer rates hardly appears coincidental. Both rates seem tied to Western lifestyles, and dietary factors are increasingly suspected as one important promoter of breast cancers. Breast-cancer risk also correlates with a variety of nondietary factors, including family medical history, income (the wealthier being more susceptible), and the age at which women bear their first child (childless or late-bearing women having the higher risk).

The same study of thirty-seven countries that associated bowel cancer with the high intake of fat and animal protein disclosed that such a diet may also be linked to breast cancer. In other studies of human populations (such as vegetarian Seventh-Day Adventists) and of animals, researchers have also tentatively connected fat intake with breast cancer incidence. The fat content of the affluent diet alters the body's balance of sex hormones, which in turn may—the theory goes—affect breast-cancer susceptibility.

Breast cancer is the most common of several kinds of cancer—including those of the prostate gland and testis among men and those of the ovary and uterus among women

—that are sometimes grouped together under the heading of
"endocrine-dependent cancers." These cancers all seem to
be influenced by the hormones secreted by the endocrine
system, and all are quite prevalent in the Western countries.
In the United States, breast cancer kills more women than
any other cancer does, while prostate cancer follows only
lung and bowel cancer as a cause of death among men.

Cancer statistics generally invite only cautious interpreta-
tion, and the international pattern in which endocrine-
dependent cancers occur is not uniform enough to allow
identification of a simple cause. Nevertheless, diet seems to
exert an influence on the incidence of these malignancies.
Dr. John W. Berg of the University of Iowa concludes:

> The most plausible hypothesis, although based on extremely incom-
> plete knowledge, is that some components of the Western high-
> protein, high-fat diet acting in early life make individuals prone to
> develop these cancers. . . . In speculation one could go as far as to
> suggest that mankind generally evolved under conditions of pru-
> dent (i.e., low-fat and protein) nutrition and that the present affluent
> diet from childhood onward may overstimulate the endocrine sys-
> tem, producing the same effect that one would obtain running a
> diesel engine on high-octane airplane fuel.

While obesity is associated with cancers of the uterine lining
and the kidney in females, the most widespread influences of
overnutrition on cancer seem to stem from the richness, not
the quantity, of food that typifies the affluent diet.[31]

No review of dietary influences on cancer would be complete without mention of the synthetic food additives and
residues with which the affluent diet is increasingly laced.
Though human-made chemicals in food probably constitute
only a small part of the diet-cancer complex, their exact
contribution to cancer rates is a conspicuous unknown, and
some unpleasant surprises are likely in store. The only cer-
tainty is that citizens in the wealthiest countries ingest a few

thousand different chemical compounds, most of which have not yet been adequately tested for links to cancer, genetic mutations, birth defects, or behavioral problems.

Suspect food additives and pesticide residues are being scrutinized in laboratories, and a few chemicals once assumed safe have been banned in one country or another. But the number of both old and new substances that need to be examined overtaxes the global testing capacity. Newly introduced additives are subjected to fairly rigorous testing, but once the food industry starts producing and people start buying a product, its removal becomes far more difficult politically. When test results are ambiguous, as they often are, and when the probability of cancerous effects on human beings appears slight, as it often does, the economic and political pressures to give a profitable product the benefit of the doubt can seem irresistible.

Some U.S. cancer researchers question whether the cancer risks associated with the high-fat, refined Western diet are clearly defined enough to warrant publicizing the potential benefits of dietary changes. A growing number, however, now recommend the adoption of a "prudent diet" to help reduce cancer risk, much as heart specialists have long recommended a battery of dietary changes without absolute proof of the benefits.[32] The strength of the case for any given food's influence on cancer remains weaker than the cardiologists' dietary case. But the argument for trying to prevent cancer through dietary changes gains appeal in view of the happy coincidence in dietary directions called for by current knowledge of both heart disease and cancer. Reduced consumption of fats, especially animal fats, and increased consumption of whole grains, fresh fruits, and vegetables, appear to be just what the doctor should order.

Outside of Scandinavia, the concept of health-centered national nutrition planning is not yet entrenched in developed countries. Fortification programs, generally high incomes, and food or income supplements have eliminated most—though by no means all—serious undernutrition in these countries. Guaranteeing adequate incomes for all the residents of developed nations could, by virtually eradicating undernutrition, provide a solid foundation for comprehensive nutritional planning designed to combat overnutrition too. But against the menace of overconsumption, most developed countries have not yet begun to fight.

Medical communities and governments both share responsibility for this failure. Most medical attention is devoted to "crises" such as heart attacks, even though these seemingly sudden attacks often reflect decades of cumulative nutritional abuse. Governments, through their agricultural, economic, and educational policies, have at best usually ignored overnutrition. At worst they have actively promoted unhealthy consumption trends. Most nutrition education addresses the dwindling deficiency problems of the past rather than the growing newer dangers of overnutrition, and key agricultural and economic decisions are made with scant regard for human health. For example, faced with mountains of surplus butter, the EEC's European Commission recently proposed taxing edible oils to make margarine as expensive as butter—in effect, to encourage higher consumption of saturated fats. In Great Britain, a recent Government White Paper on national food-production policy ignored health considerations while calling for increased output of milk, beef, and sugar beets. The Congressionally mandated involvement of the U.S. Department of Agriculture in promoting higher egg consumption in the United States provides another case in point.[33]

By subsidizing the further growth of food industries whose products are unhealthy when consumed at current levels, governments sanction the growth of those with vested interests in promoting bad health. Here, a parallel to the detrimental—and, in many countries, government-subsidized—operations of the tobacco industry might be drawn.

Many doctors and nutritionists studying overnutrition recommend the following changes for those consuming an affluent diet: fat consumption should be reduced considerably and, whenever possible, saturated fats should be replaced by unsaturated fats; cholesterol intake, especially by men, should be cut radically; sugar and salt intake should be sharply reduced; consumption of whole grains, potatoes and other starchy foods, and fresh fruits and vegetables should be increased; and, above all, personal energy intake and energy expenditure should be kept in balance, in part by calorie budgeting and in part by engaging in more physical activity. Such changes do not come easily; for many, they violate lifelong habits and strongly ingrained notions about which foods are healthful and tasty. And building exercise into a sedentary lifestyle tries most individuals. Moreover, when people revise their consumption patterns, changes will ripple through the farm and food industries as well—changes that threatened businesses cannot welcome.

A national strategy to counter overnutrition, like one to eliminate undernutrition, must involve a wide range of policies, not all of them directly linked to food and agriculture. In rich as in poor countries, the marketplace has its own set of priorities, and health is not one of them. Nutrition planning must include the development of economic incentives and institutions that encourage healthy food-production and consumption patterns.

Agricultural research, crop subsidies, taxes, meat-grading, international trade, and medical and general education rank high among the many concerns that a strategy to combat overnutrition must encompass. Since overnutrition and lack of exercise are part of the same problem, such topics as recreation and transportation policy enter into the picture as well. For example, the construction of bicycle paths rather than parking lots for urban commuters would create, among other benefits, the opportunity for regular exercise and could thereby reduce the incidence of obesity and heart disease.

Among the industrial countries, Sweden and Norway stand alone in their recent decisions to integrate modern dietary health concerns into national economic and agricultural planning. Through a vigorous public education program, the Swedish Government has worked to reduce the amount of calories, fats, sugar, and alcohol Swedes consume and to increase the amount of exercise Swedes get. The Norwegian Government has proposed to its legislature a nutrition and food policy aimed at increasing national self-sufficiency in food supplies and at cutting the mounting national toll of cardiovascular and other diet-related diseases. (In January, 1977, a U.S. Senate Committee called for a health-oriented national nutrition program, but the U.S. Government has taken no concrete steps in that direction.)[34]

The Norwegian Government has proposed establishing a broad array of subsidies, grants, price policies, and other incentives designed to stabilize meat consumption (which has been rising over the last decade); to increase fish consumption; to reduce feed-grain imports; to inculcate a preference for low-fat over whole milk; and to reverse the decline in consumption of grains, potatoes, and vegetables. The educational potential of government agencies, private organizations, and schools will be enlisted to inform Norwegians of the health implications of their eating habits. Representatives of the eight different ministries, ranging from Fisheries to Agriculture to Foreign Affairs, whose activities should be influenced by the national nutrition and food plan will meet in a coordinating body. If the nutrition plan is implemented, Norway may reduce its agricultural trade deficit and its claims on world food resources as it betters its people's health.

Representatives of threatened food industries and others

argue that strategies to alter the affluent diet cannot be justified on scientific grounds. A comprehensive review of dietary impacts on health, however, reveals a persuasive case for dietary change. The correlation of the geography of the affluent diet with the geography of the diseases it apparently promotes, together with the available experimental results, argues forcefully against this diet.

With afflictions such as coronary heart disease, whose development spans decades and is obviously influenced by many factors, the exact causative role of any one factor necessarily remains elusive. Nevertheless, that aspects of the affluent diet promote atherosclerosis and heart disease, the leading killers in the West, has been proven beyond reasonable doubt. Our understanding of dietary influences on other diseases such as cancers of the bowel, breast, and prostate is much less advanced. Yet, the dietary changes that the leading theorists of cancer causation call for are precisely those that help reduce the threats of heart disease and obesity.

Certainly more remains to be learned about diet and health, but, as Dr. D. Mark Hegsted of Harvard University observes of problems of data and proof in this field, "one does not need to know all of the answers before one can make practical recommendations." The dietary changes that doctors are prescribing involve no foreseeable health risks; quite the contrary, all evidence points to the great risks involved in clinging to our current diet. The only known risk associated with more prudent diets is that to the food industries that would be affected. But, "while these industries deserve some consideration," remarks Dr. Hegsted, "their interests cannot supersede the health interest of the population they must feed."[35]

Although the health connection is itself sufficient to justify creating programs to alter the diets of the affluent, two other considerations make such changes even more attractive. One is family food economy. Both reducing meat consumption and substituting vegetable for animal proteins save money. Grains and fresh fruits and vegetables usually cost far less than processed, pre-prepared foods and snacks that tend to be overly refined and loaded with sugar, fats, and unnecessary additives.

Second, reducing overnutrition might contribute in a small way to reducing undernutrition. Widespread moderation in the consumption of fatty grain-fed livestock products —the production of which uses up over a third of the world's grain each year—can modify the terms of the global competition between rich and poor for available food and agricultural resources. Competition for agricultural products is sometimes overt, as in the recent case of Brazilian soybeans, but it is usually manifested more subtly in the competition for products in the world marketplace and, ultimately, in the allocation of land and capital.

In the end, only individuals—who must change their behavior—can reduce overnutrition's toll. But governments have a responsibility to provide a structure of incentives and information than enhances rather than threatens the wellbeing of their populations. In the nineteenth century, as scientists became aware of the role of filth in propagating infectious disease, governments tried to provide clean water and sewage facilities. More recently, the responsibility of governments to combat undernutrition has been widely recognized. Today, our growing knowledge of the health consequences of overnutrition demands another step in the evolution of public health policies. With diet apparently a factor in more than half of all deaths in the Western countries, the new stronghold of preventive medicine must be the pantry.

5. Cancer: A Social Disease

THE COLLECTION OF DISEASES called "cancer" strikes all races and ages of people and all animal species. It has probably taken lives since human life evolved. Yet in the current century, within the last fraction of a percent of humanity's tenure, cancer has become far more prevalent than ever before. In the industrialized world, where the death toll of infectious diseases has fallen dramatically, cancer now accounts for one of every five deaths; only heart disease kills more people. In the United States alone, cancer claims a thousand lives a day. Its rising worldwide death toll already tops five million a year, and it spares neither the poor nor the rich.

Insidious, seemingly inexplicable, and more often than not fatal, cancer evokes mystery and terror to many. And, indeed, the particulars of cancer genesis baffle even the world's leading cancer scientists. Several decades and billions of dollars spent on research have greatly increased knowledge about the disease but have failed to reveal its essence. Lifesaving techniques for detecting some types of cancer early in their development have evolved, and limited gains in the success of surgical, chemical, and radiological therapies have been registered; but many kinds of malignancies still cannot be cured.

Nevertheless, ignorance of the biology of cancer does not

leave us defenseless against its ravages. Bitter experience and meticulous study have shown that cancer, like virtually all diseases, is primarily the product of interactions between organisms and their environments. Although they disagree about much, cancer researchers assert almost unanimously that the majority—probably from 70 to 90 percent—of all human cancers are induced by environmental factors and are hence theoretically preventable. Diet, cigarette smoking, and alcohol consumption; pollutants in air, water, food, and soil; toxic chemicals in workplaces or manufactured products; and exposures to sunlight and ionizing radiation all influence cancer rates. Rooted in cultural habits and technological patterns, cancer is, as one researcher put it, a "social disease."[1]

To grasp the broad array of traditional and modern social factors that promote cancer is to understand the difficulty and social conflicts that progress against cancer must entail. Not only must environmental carcinogens be identified—a painstaking, expensive process just now getting under way—but personal behavior patterns must subsequently be altered and, in some cases, economic institutions must be retooled. And personal and social inertia, bolstered by economic pressures to maintain current production and consumption patterns, can prove stronger than good sense and doctors' orders.

Yet to possess knowledge of the social origins of cancer is also to dispel the disease's aura of inevitability and immutability. Many cancer causes could be identified and then eliminated if people and polities mustered sufficient will power. Research backed up by preventive measures could push down cancer's toll even before its biological traits are fully understood, much less before any dramatic breakthroughs in cancer treatment take place.

The time that carcinogens take to work their curse complicates the task of identifying them. The damage that many

cancer agents cause does not appear until from fifteen to
forty years after the victim's exposure. To take one example,
an unusually high incidence of a rare, fatal cancer of the
chest or abdominal lining (mesothelioma) began showing up
in the 1960s among men who handled asbestos in shipyards
and elsewhere during World War II. Observant investigators
who made this particular connection firmly established the
cancerous effects of inhaled asbestos fibers. But such time
lags pose obvious problems for researchers trying to link
present-day cancers to their probable causes.

Current cancer rates reflect both the persistence of traditional (and in many cases unidentified) cultural habits that
promote cancer, and the spread of new carcinogens and cancer-promoting habits in recent decades. During the last half
century, tremendous changes in living and eating habits
have affected most of the world's people, and tens of thousands of chemical compounds—many of which are strangers
to nature and few of which have been thoroughly tested for
possible carcinogenic, mutagenic, or other harmful effects—
have been introduced into the environment. Roughly one
thousand *new* chemicals go into production *each year* in the
United States. Over the coming decades our bodies will provide clues as to how many slow-acting carcinogens have been
unleashed in the name of progress. "Our mistakes in the past
permitted many of us to be exposed to cancer agents. Our
tissues bear the imprint of these mistakes," writes Dr. Irving
J. Selikoff, a leading authority on occupationally induced cancer.[2] An acceleration of cancer's upward climb may well be
in store.

For decades, most food additives, cosmetics, and drugs
have been tested and government-regulated—though with
varying degrees of care and stringency. But until 1977, when
a landmark toxic-substances law took effect in the United
States, no law anywhere called for the systematic screening
of new industrial chemicals for potential health effects. Most

countries still do not screen and test all manufactured chemicals or force industry to monitor itself. Even the U. S. law represents no more than a first step toward coping with the health challenge of industrial chemicals.

If cancers are classified according to type and by the organs in which they appear, well over one hundred varieties —most of them rather rare—may be distinguished. In certain ways each can be considered a different disease, and almost certainly no simple cause or potential cure is common to all. Yet, all cancers are typified by the unrestrained proliferation of body cells.

When runaway cell growth remains bounded within a localized area, it usually constitutes a benign tumor, which is sometimes fatal but can usually be surgically removed. Most malignant tumors, or cancers, on the other hand, have the capacity to spread, and many eventually invade distant body parts through the bloodstream and lymphatic system. Often this dissemination (a process called metastasis), not the original tumor, brings on death. (Cancer's name itself reflects figuratively the disease's ability to divide and conquer. The Greek word for "crab" was applied by Hippocrates to the mysterious affliction that seemed to grip the body from within with crablike pincers; "cancer" is the Latin counterpart.[3])

Some malignancies spread so quickly that early detection means little. But many that are discovered before they have spread can be removed surgically or destroyed by other means, which is why early detection so often determines a cancer patient's survival prospects. Still others, perhaps deterred by the body's natural defenses, spread so slowly that their hosts may die of other causes before cancer exerts baneful effects. Mysteriously, some malignancies disappear altogether.

Just what causes cell growth to go haywire remains unknown. Certain influences and substances—such as radiation, tobacco smoke, asbestos, and vinyl chloride—definitely promote cancer genesis, but the exact causal mechanisms remain objects of conjecture at best. The individual's genetic constitution probably influences his or her chances of developing some forms of cancer. Cancer of the female breast, for instance, appears more often in some families than in others. Yet most cancers do not run along family lines. Overall, heredity appears far less important than environment as an explanation for the wide cultural variations in cancer patterns.

Viruses have long been suspected of triggering at least some kinds of cancer. Such suspicions have gained credence with the discovery that various animal species can develop a leukemia-like disease after being injected with viruses from leukemic animals. The presence of a virus in the cancerous tissues of tropical Africans who suffer from a malignancy called Burkitt's lymphoma has also been established. However, extensive research has failed to prove that viruses cause human cancer.[4]

Given the available evidence, many scientists believe that a viral role in the initiation of human leukemia, cancers of the lymph nodes, cervical cancer, and some other malignancies will eventually be established. But whatever part viruses play in cancer's origins, it almost surely differs from the role they take in initiating familiar viral diseases. Apparently, for example, some separate environmental agent triggers virally transmitted leukemia in test animals; by itself, the virus does not induce the disease. Likewise, recent evidence indicates that other factors influence the onset of those human cancers to which viruses seem linked. Chronic infection with malaria, for instance, may increase a person's susceptibility to the virus that is believed to promote Burkitt's lymphoma.[5] While it is known that many natural and synthetic chemical agents can precipitate malignancies as surely as radiation can, the function of viruses in the origin of human cancers awaits elucidation.

Some chemicals can induce cancer directly; cellular exposure to one of them may be enough to initiate a malignant tumor. Even when such carcinogens do not trigger cancer, they still may alter cells permanently, leaving them susceptible to later malignant transformation by cancer "promoters" —chemicals or even physical insults that are not carcinogenic by themselves. In contrast, some chemicals may combine with other agents to cause cancer. Excessive alcohol consumption, for example, seldom causes cancer of the mouth or larynx unless it is combined with smoking. Alcohol, most scientists therefore believe, magnifies the carcinogenic impact of some tobacco-smoke ingredient in these cases.[6] Some dietary components that are not intrinsically carcinogenic seem to encourage the body's production of carcinogens. The consumption of excessive amounts of ordinary dietary fats, for instance, may promote hormonal and digestive changes that in turn cause cancer. Some substances, such as tobacco smoke, include both direct carcinogens and agents that unleash the cancer-causing powers of other environmental influences.

Only a few dozen chemical compounds are certifiably carcinogenic in humans. Many more such agents no doubt exist: that so few substances have been proven carcinogenic in humans attests not to the rarity of carcinogens in the environment, but rather to the exceptional conditions necessary to build an airtight case against a particular agent. Establishing a statistically significant one-to-one relationship between an environmental agent and cancer poses obvious difficulties when the general population is used as the statistical base. The time lags between exposures and malignancies, and the unique constellation of chemical exposures and personal habits each person represents create unmanageable data-processing problems. For this reason, many human carcinogens have been revealed by unusual cancer patterns among workers in specialized occupations. The exposure of factory or laboratory workers to particular substances can often be measured quite accurately. Thus, when several dozen plastics workers around the world developed a rare form of liver cancer in the 1970s, the vinyl chloride to which they had all been exposed was clearly indicted.

More than a thousand substances have already been shown to induce tumors in test animals, and the number rises steadily. But for both ethical and practical reasons the effects of such chemicals on humans may never be proven. We have little choice but to assume that substances that cause cancer in animals may also imperil humans.

The current scientific understanding of the means by which chemicals induce cancer sheds some light on the problems of cancer prevention. Noncarcinogenic poisons usually stop damaging cells as soon as exposure is ended. If the poisoned person survives the exposure, healthy cells eventually replace the damaged ones. In contrast, carcinogenic agents usually appear to affect body cells irreversibly; chemical carcinogens may, many scientists now believe, damage the DNA and cause cellular mutations that persist as the cells replace themselves. In the words of Dr. W. C. Hueper, an American cancer-research pioneer, exposures of a cell to cancer-causing agents "leave a permanent carcinogenic cellular imprint which makes it more susceptible to the effects of subsequent exposures." Contacts with a carcinogen, even if separated by long intervals, can thus have an additive impact, gradually increasing the probability that cancer will ensue. Each malignancy, writes Dr. John Cairns, may be "the end result of several mutational steps that may have taken place at any time in the patient's life." While some cancers result from a brief contact with a powerful carcinogen in the distant past, others seem to be caused by a lifetime of intermittent or chronic exposures to low levels of carcinogens.

Along with the lengthy gap between exposure to carcinogens and the advent of cancer, this cumulative effect may help explain the high prevalence of cancer among the aged; naturally, the probability that accumulated cancer-promoting mutations will reach a critical point rises with age.[7]

If the effects of carcinogenic exposures are irreversible and cumulative, our approach to cancer prevention must differ from that underlying the regulation of more familiar toxic materials. For most poisons, a permissible exposure level is established below which no (or only slight) harm to humans is believed to occur. But because cancer-related cell damage is irreparable, time must also be taken into account. One week's low-level exposure to a particular agent may itself fail to cause cancer, but to this must be added the potential cumulative impact of any other exposures to the carcinogen in a person's lifetime, as well as the effects that other agents may have on the same cells. Clearly, to be effective, cancer-prevention campaigns must aim at reducing the lifetime burden of carcinogens to which people are exposed.

Identifying the environmental causes of cancer has been a slow process. Inherently difficult, the task is also relatively thankless and has not received the resources that an all-out effort needs. Already, however, enough is known about many important cancer-inducing agents to allow individuals and societies to reduce cancer's future toll substantially. Acquiescence to unhealthy behavior and production patterns, as much as a lack of knowledge, insures that cancer rates will remain high in coming decades.

Far and away the largest single proven cause of cancer in the world today is cigarette smoke. Because of the unprecedented global popularity of cigarettes in the twentieth century, lung cancer is now a spreading worldwide scourge. Relatively rare only a century ago, it now leads all other cancers in the industrial countries as a cause of death. Moreover, the current upward trend in total cancer deaths in some countries, including the United States, largely reflects rising lung-cancer mortality. Personal smoking habits—combined sometimes with exposure to radiation, asbestos, or other pollutants—unquestionably underlie current lung-cancer trends.

People who smoke habitually for decades suffer at least a tenfold increase in their odds of dying from lung cancer, while heavy smokers' risks can run twenty times higher than those of nonsmokers. Tobacco smoke also causes or promotes cancers of the mouth, throat, bladder, esophagus, and pancreas. According to the American Cancer Society, cigarette smoking is responsible for 15 to 20 percent of all cancers in the United States.[8]

How civilization arrived at the curious present state of affairs, how the deadly cigarette came to be subsidized by governments, advertised by companies, and purchased daily by hundreds of millions of people is a story worth its own chapter (See Chapter 6). Whatever the forces that keep the smoking habit so prevalent, a war on cancer is necessarily a war on smoking.

A second major category of cancer causes involves diet. Although this contention is not yet backed by solid proof, all dietary factors together may outstrip even tobacco as a worldwide contributor to cancer. Current evidence, says Dr. Ernst L. Wynder, president of the American Health Foundation, suggests that diet is related to "as much as 50 percent of all cancers in women and one-third of all cancers in men."[9]

The public often thinks about the link between diet and cancer only in terms of chemical food additives. But while synthetic additives pose real enough problems, research over the last quarter century is pointing to other, as yet only dimly perceived dietary factors that may exert a far weightier influence on cancer rates. Under suspicion are some concerns scarcely even considered by most nutritionists in the past:

the degree to which foods are processed, the role of fats in the diet, food storage practices, deficiencies or surpluses of trace elements and vitamins, and even the type of preparation some foods receive.

The high-fat, highly refined diet of the world's more affluent countries, many researchers suspect, promotes several important kinds of malignancies, including cancers of the bowel, breast, and prostate gland (See Chapter 4). At the same time, some unknown ingredient of the affluent diet seems to be reducing the incidence of stomach cancer. Over the last half century, stomach cancer rates have declined markedly in the United States and in several European countries, though stomach cancer remains one of the more prevalent malignancies even in these countries. Recently, stomach cancer incidence has also begun to decline in some countries with exceptionally high rates, including Japan, where the incidence is the world's highest. This global decline constitutes one of the most pronounced cancer trends in the century and is almost certainly diet-related; yet its cause eludes cancer researchers. At work in a world fraught with pernicious cancer mysteries, these benevolent unknown forces offer some solace.

Several factors have been isolated as possible contributors to the exceptional incidence of stomach cancer in Japan. A national penchant for dried, salted fish and pickled vegetables is one; many believe that the nitrosamines, known carcinogens that these foods often contain, are the main culprits. Asbestos residues on talc-coated white rice, without which no Japanese meal is complete, could also promote cancer. The mountains of smoked fish consumed each year in Japan may also prove cancerous; they contain chemicals called polycyclic aromatic hydrocarbons that have long been known to be carcinogenic in other contexts. Internationally, all populations that consume large amounts of smoked fish have high rates of stomach cancer. But no single factor has been identified as common to all regions in which stomach cancer is prevalent.[10]

Much recent speculation has centered on nitrosamines as major causes of stomach cancer. Consuming these dangerous chemicals directly poses some problem, but probably more important are the chemical combinations in food and water, the methods of food treatment, and the overall dietary patterns that allow the body to manufacture nitrosamines. Nitrite, which can combine with certain food or drug components to form nitrosamines, is often formed naturally from salivary nitrates. But the level of nitrite in the body may be influenced by the amounts of nitrite or nitrate consumed. The water supplies in parts of England, Japan, Israel, Chile, and Colombia where stomach cancer incidence is high are nitrate rich; and high natural nitrate levels in the soils of these regions may mean that locally produced food has heavy concentrations of nitrates too. The use of fertilizers containing nitrates can also boost the nitrate content of food. Moreover, fish and cured-meat products often contain small amounts of nitrates and nitrites added as preservatives.[11]

The geographic and cultural patchwork of esophageal-cancer zones is even more perplexing than the erratic stomach-cancer pattern. The incidence of esophageal cancer varies wildly among countries, within countries, and according to the victim's sex and race within specific regions. Unfortunately, esophageal malignancies have become more common in several countries over the last few decades.

Especially bewildering to scientists is the distribution of esophageal cancer in Central Asia, where—Persian writings from 1100 A.D. inform us—this affliction is no newcomer. Exceptionally high rates occur near the Caspian coast of Iran, but among groups living within a three-hundred-mile stretch the incidence varies as much as thirtyfold for women and sixfold for men. The zone of high risk encompasses northern China and the Soviet republics of Turkmenia, Kazakhstan, and Uzbekistan as well as Iran, where an office of the U. N.'s International Agency for Research on Cancer has been established to investigate this curious cancer mosaic.[12]

In Africa, esophageal cancer also appears in unusual geographic patterns. While the disease is rare in West Africa, several areas of southern and eastern Africa have experienced a dramatic rise in esophageal cancer over the last 40 years—a rise comparable to the rise of lung cancer in the industrial countries. The most promising explanation put forward so far is that the increased incidence of this cancer is linked to the increased consumption of maize-based beer in this century. Some unidentified product of the fermentation process may be carcinogenic.[13]

Associations between alcohol consumption and esophageal cancer have been established in the United States, France, Puerto Rico, and Northern Europe.[14] Alcohol consumption alone boosts the risk, as does cigarette smoking alone, but the combination of heavy drinking and smoking packs a particularly deadly wallop. In the United States, moderate smokers who drink heavily are twenty-five times more likely than nondrinking smokers to develop esophageal cancer. Although overall U.S. rates for this cancer are low, black Americans have suffered a sharp, unexplained rise in the incidence of esophageal cancer since 1940. Especially hard-hit are northern urban blacks.

Alcohol consumption can damage the mouth and throat as well as the esophagus. Heavy drinkers in the United States are from two to six times more likely than nondrinkers to contract mouth and throat cancers, with the precise risk dependent on smoking habits. Alcohol and tobacco consumption together are responsible for three-fourths of all oral cavity cancers in U. S. males. Alcoholics develop cancer of the larynx far more frequently than do nonalcoholics—again, smoking multiplies the risk. They also are more likely to contract liver cancer, which often follows upon the heels of cirrhosis, an inflammatory liver disease that afflicts mainly heavy drinkers.

Both human disease patterns and the results of experiments on animals suggest that alcohol itself seldom causes cancer, but rather enhances the carcinogenic impact of other agents. What is more, two-thirds of all cancers associated with combinations of alcohol and tobacco consumption could be prevented by eliminating smoking.[15]

One important dietary carcinogen was discovered quite by chance following the mysterious deaths of 100,000 turkeys and ducks in the United Kingdom in 1960. A powerful natural carcinogen that often finds its way into human food was at fault. Aflatoxin, which is produced by a mold that can grow on peanuts, grains, and other foods, has achieved a dubious distinction as the most potent known chemical carcinogen in rats. Aflatoxin has also been linked to human cancer.

The mold that produces aflatoxin thrives under sustained, moist warmth and is therefore most common in tropical countries. The discovery of aflatoxin's deadly power and the subsequent analysis of marketed foods for aflatoxin content over the last decade may finally make fathomable the high incidence of liver cancer in patches of the tropics. Aflatoxin contamination has already been correlated with liver cancer rates in parts of Kenya, Mozambique (where the world's highest incidence of liver cancer is found), Swaziland, the Ivory Coast, Thailand, and the Philippines.[16] Under the right conditions, aflatoxin can accumulate in foods in temperate zones too. Since its presence in internationally traded products is always possible, food inspectors everywhere are being forced to redouble their vigilance.

In many ways, nutritional influences on cancer present an even greater scientific and social challenge than does the tobacco-cancer connection. As the foregoing review makes clear, the study of diet and cancer produces no single conspicuous villain—no dietary equivalent of the cigarette. Indeed, each culture's unique mix of dietary habits leads to a specific group of diet-related cancers. Tracking down all the possible links and then eliminating the harmful foods or consumption patterns wherever possible will require perseverence, patience, and cultural changes.

The ultraviolet radiation in sunlight is another important contributor to cancer whose impact is strongly influenced by personal behavior. In the United States and many other countries, skin cancer is so common and nearly always so readily cured that many statistical studies of cancer incidence ignore it. A small proportion of skin cancers, however, involve melanoma, a fast-growing, often deadly tumor that kills five thousand Americans each year. The 300,000 skin cancer cases reported annually in the United States equal in number those of all other malignancies combined.

Sunlight promotes skin cancer, especially among light-skinned people. The longer or the more intense the exposure to solar radiation, the greater the influence. Thus, the closer to the equator that light-skinned people live, the higher their rates of skin cancer.[17] Similarly, sunbathing increases the dose of solar radiation, and many scientists feel that the increased incidence of melanoma is partly a consequence of the widespread social preference for tanned skin.

Because sunlight and skin cancer are connected, Westernization may be exacting an unexpected price in the Middle East. According to Dr. N. T. Racoveanu of the World Health Organization, the transition from traditional robes and head coverings to Western-style dress in this sun-drenched region is bound to boost the incidence of skin cancer.[18] Fear that global skin cancer rates will rise also underlies recent scientific concern about the potential depletion of the atmosphere's ozone layer, which partially filters the ultraviolet rays that promote skin cancer (See Chapter 7).

Far more potent than solar radiation is ionizing radiation,

the kind involved in nuclear reactions and medical X rays. Studies of the human survivors of the atomic bomb blasts in Hiroshima and Nagasaki, of miners and laboratory workers exposed to radiation, and of test animals have established that ionizing radiation causes cancer and genetic mutations. Indeed, as knowledge of the dangers has grown throughout this century, the national and international standards for "permissible" exposures to radiation have been steadily and drastically reduced. But the precise danger involved in exposure to a particular dosage of radiation, and the hazards attending long-term exposure to low levels of radiation, remain unknown.[19]

In developed countries, most ionizing radiation comes from nature itself (cosmic rays and radioactive materials in the earth) and from medical and dental X rays. Radioactive exposures attributable to nuclear fallout are comparatively small, and known exposures to radiation leaking from nuclear power facilities smaller still. Yet any potential increases in human-caused radioactive exposures deserve concern. While they cannot agree about the absolute size of the risks involved, most scientists studying radiation hazards agree that *all* exposures are probably harmful to some degree.[20]

The benefits of a particular exposure to radiation need to be balanced with the health risks it entails. The value of an accurate diagnosis of, say, a possible broken leg clearly outweighs the extremely slight danger posed by a properly performed X ray. On the other hand, fetal exposure to X rays, we now know, involves a cancer risk seldom worth taking. (According to Sir Richard Doll, 5 to 10 percent of all childhood cancers in Western Europe and North America during the 1950s and 1960s probably resulted from X ray exposures of pregnant women.) Deciding whether or not to take a particular risk can be a tricky and imprecise business. In a controversial 1976 decision, the U. S. National Cancer Institute withdrew its support for a breast-tumor detection program involving the mass X ray screening of women under age fifty. The (disputed) fear was that the screening program might produce as many breast cancers decades later as it discovered today.[21]

In 1964, a WHO Expert Committee noted "the need for massive reduction of medical doses" of radiation. Yet to this day, medical exposures often exceed the necessary intensity. Even in more technically advanced countries, many people receive unnecessarily high X rays from faulty equipment or careless operators, and X rays are often taken when they are not needed. For the small proportion of poor-country populations that has access to modern clinics, conditions are generally worse still; malfunctioning equipment and overexposures are commonplace.[22]

Producing electricity with nuclear power has added to society a new source of ionizing radiation. If the more grandiose plans for nuclear power were to materialize—which now appears unlikely—the globe would within a few decades be dotted with thousands of nuclear power plants and reprocessing facilities, and crisscrossed by transportation routes for radioactive fuels and wastes. As the supply of uranium fuel dwindled, countries would likely begin to construct "breeder" reactors that create more reactor fuel than they consume. Plutonium, the fuel breeders create, is one of the deadliest substances known; moreover, it remains hazardous for hundreds of thousands of years and is a basic ingredient of nuclear bombs.

Even in the absence of human or mechanical errors, the day-to-day operations of the nuclear power system—including uranium mining and milling, power-plant operations, nuclear fuel reprocessing, and transporting and storing of radioactive fuels and wastes—involve the slight leakage of various radioactive materials into the environment. If nuclear power production were to expand as much as its proponents hope, by the turn of the century such "planned" pollution would probably cause anywhere from several hundreds to tens of thousands of cancer deaths and genetic mutations annually worldwide. The size of the toll would depend on the magnitude of the leaks and the toxicity of the various radioactive materials involved.[23]

Unplanned releases of radioactivity have nuclear power critics most worried. No complex system is accident-free, and no human is infallible. The chances of an accidental nuclear explosion at a power plant are infinitesimally small, but an accident involving the release of radiation is more conceivable. Already, with fewer than two hundred reactors in operation for a relatively brief period, several near-catastrophes have set nuclear critics and those who live near reactors on edge. Transporting and storing radioactive materials presents its own problems; to date, tons of weapons-grade materials simply cannot be accounted for in the United States.[24] Nor can the prospects of deliberate theft, nuclear weapons proliferation, or the sabotage of power plants be lightly dismissed.

The health and social consequences of nuclear power should be weighed against the long-term consequences of alternate energy futures. Fossil fuel-based energy systems carry health risks of their own, as the analysis of air pollution's hazards in Chapter 7 makes clear. But comparatively benign energy sources, including solar and biological energy systems, now appear workable. These sources pose few direct health hazards and none of the imponderable dangers of a nuclear-powered world.[25]

Individuals can quit smoking or flee smoke-filled places. To some degree they can also control their diets and regulate their exposures to sunlight. But pollutants such as radioactive fallout present another kind of challenge; broader social forces determine individuals' exposures. Similarly, cancer-promoting medical drugs represent a hazard whose control depends on more than personal choice. In theory, individuals can determine their own medical treatment; in practice, few do. Few laymen have the knowledge or the self-confidence to question the propriety of a drug prescription; most place themselves at their doctors' mercy.

Drugs are biologically active substances by definition, and many produce unwanted side effects. Both governmental regulations and promulgated medical ethics aim at keeping dangerous drugs off the market except in those cases in which the benefits of a particular, carefully circumscribed use outbalance the health risks such use entails. For example, although certain immuno-suppressive drugs may cause cancer, life-saving kidney transplants cannot succeed without them. Unfortunately, however, inadequate testing (especially for subtle long-term effects) and, occasionally, inadequate governmental regulation have sometimes resulted in drug-induced tragedies. The Thalidomide scandal of the early 1960s, in which pregnant women in Europe were sold a sedative that turned out to cause birth defects, provides a well known case in point.

Drug testing and drug regulation have come a long way since the 1920s, when, according to the book *100,000,000 Guinea Pigs,* a charlatan named William J. A. Bailey could freely peddle Radithor—a deadly concoction of radioactive salts and water—as a cure for 160 diseases and conditions. Then the agonizing death of one gullible customer was vividly described in *Time* magazine.[26] Today, such willful deception is less common, and the use of a drug with proven carcinogenic or other dangerous properties will not long go unregulated. Yet gross mishandling of possibly carcinogenic medicines by negligent doctors and government officials may still occur, as the recent story of DES (diethylstilbestrol) illustrates.

Since the 1940s, the estrogen DES has been prescribed to between 500,000 and two million pregnant women in the

United States in the mistaken belief that the drug helps prevent spontaneous abortion. A sudden rash of rare vaginal cancers in the 1970s among more than one hundred young women whose mothers had taken DES during pregnancy about two decades earlier revealed the cancer hazard that DES poses. The treatment given this issue by some members of the medical community has been criminally lax. As National Cancer Institute doctors Robert Hoover and Joseph Fraumeni pointed out in 1975, "In the early 1960s DES was still being given to a surprisingly large number of pregnant women years after its efficacy in preventing spontaneous abortion had been disproved. Even with the recent publicity about carcinogenic hazards to the fetus, within the past year prescriptions for DES were still being written for pregnant women."[27] Among other things, the DES scandal points to the dangers of sexual homogeneity in the male-dominated medical, pharmaceutical, and regulatory professions.

Carcinogenic industrial chemicals constitute another category of potential cancer sources whose production and use the individual cannot control. In the world's more "advanced" countries, living even for a few days without eating, drinking, or breathing any of the chemicals created and dispersed by industrial society would be virtually impossible. Fortunately, all indications are that only a small fraction of the tens of thousands of synthetic chemicals now permeating daily life are carcinogenic or otherwise hazardous. The challenge is to identify the unsafe ones—preferably before their use is widespread—and then to minimize or eliminate human contact with them.

Asbestos in ceiling insulation, arsenic in the air, chloroform in cosmetics and drinking water, PCBs in fish and mothers' milk, vinyl chloride in factories and their effluents—the list of recent "revelations" lengthens almost weekly. Each time it is discovered that a familiar substance is hazardous or that a known hazard has crept into a new corner of our habitat, the public registers shock. After a point, however, such "surprises" come to appear predestined by our ways of doing certain things. In a call for legislation to make screening new industrial chemicals for health hazards mandatory, Russell Train, then chief of the Environmental Protection Agency, observed:

> There are today more than 30,000 chemicals in actual commercial production; every year, this list grows by some 1,000 new compounds. Of the more than two million known chemicals, only a few thousand have been tested for carcinogenicity and—aside from those used in food additives, drugs and pesticides—only a few hundred have been adequately tested. We know, in fact, very little about the health effects even of the 30,000 chemicals already in commercial production. We have no way of systematically screening the chemicals that do go into production; we have no way of knowing precisely which chemicals go into production every year. In other words, we not only don't know whether what's going out there is dangerous—we don't even know what's going out there.
>
> We have, however, learned one thing: it's what we don't know that can really hurt us, even kill us.[28]

Potentially dangerous chemicals are most widely disseminated in the more developed countries, but Africans, Asians, and Latin Americans are not altogether free of such risks. Refineries and factories in poor countries can expose workers and those in the vicinity of a plant to known carcinogens just as similar facilities in rich countries do.[29] In fact, the lack of skilled scientists to serve as industrial "watchdogs" in poor countries often means that working conditions and pollution discharges are less well monitored and regulated than they tend to be in rich ones. Likewise, pesticide residues in food, unsafe drugs, and harmful cosmetics are less apt to be carefully watched and firmly controlled by governments in developing countries.

One generation ago, few of the materials of everyday life were tested for toxicity, and information on the trends and global distribution of cancers—information that could have provided telltale clues about dangerous habits and chemicals —was scarce. A lethal smoke ring had to girdle the globe, for example, before antismoking campaigns gathered force; not until midcentury did hard evidence suggest that cigarettes had become a major cause of cancer. Once industrial processes and social habits become entrenched, of course, altering, discouraging, or removing them becomes far more difficult and controversial than prior prevention would have been.

The present-day escalation in laboratory testing of materials for carcinogenicity, though still inadequate, is shifting the experimental burden from unwitting people to the laboratory animals on which, most agree, it belongs. While far from perfect, the testing procedures used today are reliable enough to warrant their application to many more chemicals than have yet been evaluated. Thorough tests using animals often cost well over $100,000 per chemical and take two to four years. But cancer's toll is not cheap either; its direct and indirect annual economic costs total tens of billions of dollars, and the personal anguish to victims and their families costs more than dollars can tell.

The tremendous financial burden involved in the extensive testing of chemicals for cancer may be lightened somewhat by new quick and inexpensive testing procedures that make use of bacteria or even cultured cells rather than mammals. Such tests are not totally reliable, cancer specialists warn; but the tests may be useful as an initial screening technique, to be backed up when necessary with full-scale animal tests.[30]

Laboratory tests and detective-like investigations of cancer variations among different populations are together revealing ever more of the causes of human cancer. The most difficult challenge in cancer prevention over the coming decades will probably not be identifying carcinogens but

reducing human contacts with such agents and altering cancer-promoting cultural patterns.

Irreversible and additive, the effects of carcinogenic exposures present special problems in the regulation of cancer-
causing chemicals. Ordinarily, a "safe" exposure level to a
toxic substance is determined and then imposed on industry.
But, as a blue-ribbon panel of U.S. cancer researchers reported in 1970, "no level of exposure to a chemical carcinogen should be considered toxicologically insignificant for
man. For carcinogenic agents a 'safe level for man' cannot be
established by application of our present knowledge. The
concept of 'socially acceptable risk' represents a more realistic notion." Moreover, the panel went on to note, "it has
become increasingly obvious that the hazard from a single
chemical carcinogen cannot be evaluated out of context of
the total environmental exposure. Estimation of the 'cumulative carcinogenic dose' resulting from all possible chemical
carcinogens or even from all sources of a single type or class
of chemical carcinogens is presently impossible."[31] Calculat-
ing the "socially acceptable risk" of a substance whose production and sale may involve millions of dollars and thousands of jobs, but which may contribute to an unknown
number of human cancers, is obviously no mere mathemati-
cal task.

Tobacco use and dietary patterns are far less amenable
than suspect industrial chemicals to governmental regulation or banishment. In choosing lifestyles, individuals go a
long way toward determining their own odds with cancer.
According to Dr. John Higginson, Director of the International Agency for Research on Cancer, a male in a developed nation "who lives in the country, does not smoke,
eats and drinks with moderation, and reduces his exposure
to sunlight may reduce his risk of cancer by at least 30–40
percent or possibly more according to the country in
which he lives. The corresponding figures for females are
somewhat less."[32]

Still, governments do influence the habits of individuals and thus have a responsibility to make those influences as beneficial as possible. To do so, governments can ensure that all are made to understand the probable risks of various lifestyles, thus promoting the freest possible choice even in a social climate conditioned by commercial messages that are hardly rooted in medical wisdom. Governments can remove subsidies from unhealthy products such as tobacco, alter regulations that influence dietary patterns, and generally influence the evolution of institutions that promote or discourage dangerous habits.

If smoking were curtailed, if eating habits were made to reflect what we know about cancer, if more chemicals were tested for carcinogenic potential and the uses of more suspicious agents were cut back, the incidence of cancer would plummet. Dr. John Cairns calculates that "if by the appropriate public-health measures the incidence of each kind of cancer were reduced to the lowest level observed anywhere in the world, the overall incidence of cancer would be reduced at least tenfold. That is roughly equivalent to the reduction in mortality from infectious diseases that has been achieved in the past fifty years."[33]

Cairns' calculation postulates a new dispensation, an ideal world in which virtually all environmental causes of all forms of cancer can be both identified and eliminated from human life. Such idealism remains, of course, chimerical. Experience proves that self-destructive habits such as smoking can hold their own against the clearest and most damning scientific evidence. Dietary cancer-promoters may be too numerous, complex, or culturally ingrained to eliminate totally. Over time, the study of unusual cancer patterns and the laboratory screening of substances will no doubt unveil many of the carcinogens that permeate modern life. But so long as people live in a complex industrial society chock full of substances nature would disown, some cancerous influences are bound to evade the cleverest controls.

The cancer trends of the next quarter century have already been set in motion. But the more distant future is clay in our hands. Personal and societal decisions made today inconspicuously but surely determine the social role cancer will play at the turn of the century and beyond. The smoking habits today's children learn from advertisers or their parents; the diets on which they are raised; the chemicals they eat, drink, or breathe—all will influence their health in adulthood.

6. The Unnatural History of Tobacco

WHEN ACCOSTING A TOURIST, a street waif in Cairo is as apt to beg for a cigarette as for coins. In China, a country renowned for its preventive health-care campaigns, national leaders chain-smoke as they preside over the world's largest tobacco industry. More than a decade after the U.S. Government declared smoking to be an undeniable health hazard, four out of ten American men and three out of ten American women smoke—and the federal Department of Agriculture spends $50 million a year supporting the tobacco industry.

How is it, then, that such a harmful product has become so firmly entrenched in daily life the world over? That tobacco occupies good farmland in India while peasants starve nearby? That the cigarette merchants are allowed to use Madison Avenue's wiliest marketing techniques to cajole youngsters into a lifetime of smoking? Like a dime novel, the tale of the three-cent cigarette is a tale of intrigue, corporate power, and governmental hypocrisy; of human pleasure, addiction, and premature death.

"This vice will always be condemned and always clung to," wrote the Italian physician Bernardino Ramazzini in 1713 of tobacco use. Trying to figure out why Italian tobacco work-

ers prized their jobs despite the severe head and stomach
ailments tobacco dust inflicted upon them, Ramazzini made
another observation of equal present-day weight when he
noted that "the sweet smell of gain makes the smell of tobacco less perceptible and less offensive to those workers."[1]

Although the medical case against smoking has been con-
clusively established only within the last quarter century,
tobacco has had powerful opponents, as well as powerful
champions, almost from the moment sixteenth-century ex-
plorers gave Europe its first whiff. Yet from the beginning,
social fashions, the lure of profits, and the association of tobacco with relaxation have all helped propagate its use.
Today, despite the medical community's consensus and ex-
hortations, the smoking habit continues to spread in most of
the world. Indeed, many countries are just now entering the
era of tobacco-induced disease and death.

Native Americans were the first tobacco smokers, but
their European conquerors turned smoking and other forms
of tobacco use into global habits. Sir Walter Raleigh, the
colorful favorite of Queen Elizabeth's court, popularized
smoking in England during the late sixteenth century; the
practice caught on fast, and early orders for tobacco were
filled in Spain's New World colonies. Upon Elizabeth's death
in 1603, however, British rule fell to James I, who found
Raleigh's smoking habit as objectionable as he found the
courtier's politics. (James eventually beheaded Raleigh for
political reasons, but one nineteenth-century writer claimed
that smokers could consider Raleigh "the first martyr in their
cause."[2])

James declared that tobacco use was unhealthy, unholy,
and altogether unbefitting a civilized society. He concluded
his famous *Counter-Blaste to Tobacco,* published in 1604, by
characterizing smoking as "A custom lothsome to the eye,
hatefull to the Nose, harmefull to the braine, dangerous to
the Lungs, and in the blacke stinking fume thereof, neerest

resembling the horrible Stigian smoke of the pit that is bot-
tomelesse."

Even as James fumed, other people were making extrava-
gant claims about the salubrious powers of tobacco smoke.
Some doctors prescribed smoking as an antidote to colds and
fevers, and some even believed that inhaled smoke might
ward off the plague. During the plague year of 1603, all the
schoolboys at Eton "were obliged to smoak in the school
every morning," reported a certain Tom Rogers, who also
said that he never received a harsher whipping than the one
he suffered one morning as punishment for not smoking.[3]

Despite the antismoking campaign conducted by several
of James' successors, and the opposition of Emperor Jehangir
in India, tobacco use quickly spread throughout Europe and
then, through commerce and the tentacles of the colonial
system, to the world. As one pipe-lover waxed in 1895 over
tobacco's spread, "prince and peasant alike yielded to its
mild but irresistable sway." In eighteenth-century Italy,
Ramazzini reported, tobacco was smoked or inhaled by
"women as well as men and even children," and its purchase
was "reckoned among the daily expenses of a family."[4]

Spreading fast and far, tobacco became one of the most
widely diffused artifacts in modern history. When a Stone
Age group, the Tasaday, was recently discovered in a Philip-
pine rain forest, the group's total unfamiliarity with tobacco
was regarded by anthropologists as remarkable evidence of
the group's long isolation. (Unknowingly showing good sense,
the Tasaday made a point of returning the tobacco their
discoverers offered them, while keeping gifts of knives, cloth,
bows and arrows, rice, and salt.)[5]

The spreading demand and, hence, growing commercial
market for tobacco in sixteenth- and seventeenth-century
Europe spurred the emergence of a lucrative industry. British colonists settled in Virginia expecting to cash in on the
New World's precious metals, lumber, furs, and fish; instead,

they learned that only tobacco exports could keep their colony afloat. Virginia was nearly abandoned in 1614, but tobacco soon brought prosperity to the colony. It eventually became the economic backbone of the South Atlantic colonies despite the strong opposition of the English king and even of the founding colonial companies to reliance on this crop.[6] The "sweet smell of gain" proved a potent force indeed; and, although tobacco no longer dominates the economies of these states as totally as it once did, the tobacco industry still wields considerable force in these and other tobacco-producing areas of the world. And today, the tobacco market has a new dimension. On top of traditional public demand for tobacco, the industry's scientific manipulation of images and generation of "needs" work to *create* an ever larger market.

The popularity of one or another form of tobacco use has varied with changing notions of vogue. In eighteenth-century England, for example, the practice of sniffing snuff all but replaced the smoking habit for nearly a hundred years. In the current century, however, cigarettes have nearly everywhere edged out pipes, cigars, snuff, and chewing tobacco as the medium of choice. Unfortunately, cigarette smoking also happens to be the most dangerous form of tobacco use.

Skillful marketing by the cigarette companies undoubtedly helped sell the public on cigarettes during the early twentieth century. But the power of advertising alone cannot account for the symbolic value with which cigarettes have been invested. Simple tubes of tobacco have come to represent modernity, savoir-faire, and, in the minds of children who for decades have plunked down nickels for candy cigarettes and bubblegum cigars, adulthood. Hollywood may be one culprit. Humphrey Bogart would not be Humphrey Bogart without a cigarette drooping from his mouth, and the example of Lauren Bacall asking "Got a match?" helped identify cigarettes as the essential social crutch. Even Bogart's death from esophageal cancer could not dampen the mystique of cigarettes, their aura of sweet success and glamour that movies continue to foster. In contemporary Soviet films, comments the satirical Moscow magazine *Krokodil,* "when an actor handsome like Apollo . . . takes a cigarette into his fingers, it isn't accidental. It means the time has come for a director to demonstrate that his character can also think."[7]

Only quite recently has the compilation of an awesome medical case against cigarettes begun to tarnish the social sheen of smoking. Many thoughtful doctors had long suspected that cigarettes promote ill health, but proof of the risks eluded researchers until the mid-twentieth century. As recently as the early 1900s, cigarette advertisers could claim with impunity that their products actually promoted better health.

A startling jump in the number of lung-cancer deaths in North America and Europe provided the first widely accepted proof of smoking's hazards. Lung cancer was rare everywhere in the nineteenth century, but in the twentieth it rapidly emerged as the leading cause of cancer deaths in many countries. By 1950, studies in England and the United States had shown an exceptionally close correlation between personal smoking habits and lung-cancer incidence. By 1953, the prestigious *New England Journal of Medicine* could characterize the evidence linking cigarettes and lung cancer as "so strong as to be considered proof within the everyday meaning of the word." Then, in 1954, British and U.S. researchers independently established that smokers have a markedly higher *overall* death rate in any given year than nonsmokers do. Yet, defying reason, more and more people picked up the habit. Women and teenagers—who had lagged far behind adult men in adopting the practice—and the wealthier classes in Africa, Asia, and Latin America all joined the ranks of the smokers.[8]

In the early 1960s, two landmark public documents that crystalized the evidence on smoking's health effects caused something of a turning point in the social history of tobacco. Both a report released in 1962 by the Royal College of Physicians of London and one published in 1964 by the Surgeon General of the United States presented the massive and growing medical case against tobacco.[9] These and other similar documents prompted some governments to educate people about the hazards of smoking and to place partial restrictions on cigarette advertising. As a result, the word on smoking's risks has now been fairly effectively disseminated within at least the industrial countries. Most people, even most heavy smokers, realize that they are likely shortening their lives as they smoke.

The most widely recognized health consequence of smoking is probably the heightened risk of lung cancer—which unnecessarily takes hundreds of thousands of lives around the world each year. Lung cancer deaths are much more common among men than among women, but the gap is narrowing as the legacy of the rise in female smoking a quarter century back begins to make itself felt.

Past studies have shown that cigarette smokers are at least ten times more likely than nonsmokers to develop lung malignancies. (Those smoking newer low-tar cigarettes may face somewhat lower risks.) Many researchers feel that tobacco is responsible for eight or nine of every ten lung cancers. Combinations of tobacco smoke with air pollution or with toxic substances in workplaces undoubtedly add to the cancer tolls; tobacco smoke and certain other pollutants operate together to multiply disease risks dramatically. For example, asbestos workers who smoke have ninety-two times the lung cancer risk of men who neither smoke nor come into regular contact with asbestos. But cigarettes alone almost certainly account for most lung cancer cases. Dr. Gio B. Gori of the U.S. National Cancer Institute estimates that people smoking two packs of cigarettes a day for a year expose their lungs to nineteen times more benzpyrene—just one of the possible carcinogens in cigarette smoke—then they would by breathing the polluted air of Los Angeles for a year.[10]

Other organs and tissues besides the lungs become especially cancer-prone in chronic smokers. Smoking pipes or cigars, as well as puffing on cigarettes, raises a person's odds of developing cancers of the mouth, throat, and voice box, particularly if the smoker is a heavy drinker. Cigarette smoking also multiplies the smoker's chances of developing cancer in the esophagus, pancreas, and bladder. But, more frequent and more deadly than these other malignancies, lung cancer poses a greater threat to the smoker's life than all the other smoking-induced cancers together. After considering the entire spectrum of cancers and what is known about their causes, the president of the American Cancer Society recently stated: "Wipe out smoking and you eliminate some 15 to 20 percent of *all* cancer deaths in this and many other countries."[11]

The publicity that the connection between cigarette smoking and cancer has received is well deserved, but far more deaths arising from cigarette smoking involve coronary heart disease—the leading killer in most developed countries —than cancer. Smoking clearly taxes the heart; a middle-aged American man who smokes is twice as likely as a non-smoking man to suffer a heart attack. Female smokers, too, experience a significant increase in their heart attack odds. Moreover, smoking combines with other major risk factors, such as high blood cholesterol and high blood pressure, to multiply manyfold the heart disease risk for both sexes.[12]

While the intense search for carcinogens in tobacco smoke has exposed tars as agents provocateurs, research on the heart and circulatory system suggests that another smoke constituent, carbon monoxide, influences coronary death rates. When men with heart conditions are experimentally exposed to heavy carbon-monoxide concentrations, the chest pains of angina pectoris are set off by less exercise than usual and persist longer than usual after exertion has stopped. Coronary patients have a limited capacity to supply their hearts with rich blood; carbon monoxide exposure further reduces this capacity by impeding the transfer of oxygen from the blood to body tissue. Thus, carbon monoxide pollution (and possibly nicotine inhalation too) places an added strain upon the heart and increases the likelihood that those already susceptible to heart attacks will experience them. Chronic heavy exposure to carbon monoxide may also promote the development of atherosclerosis, which, over time, can lead to heart attacks. Autopsy studies show that lifelong smokers tend to have more severe coronary atherosclerosis than nonsmokers do, and animals exposed to carbon monoxide develop higher blood-cholesterol counts and more atherosclerosis than unexposed animals do.[13]

Not surprisingly, cigarette smokers take on tremendously increased risks of developing long-term respiratory ailments such as chronic bronchitis and emphysema. Charged with killing tens of thousands and with disabling far more each year in Europe and North America alone, these diseases have emerged as recognized public health problems only over the last century. The twin onslaught on the lungs posed by industrial air pollution and tobacco smoke undoubtedly explains why chronic respiratory diseases are growing in frequency. But cigarettes seem to be the major contributor. Cigarette smokers are five times as likely as nonsmokers to die from chronic bronchitis or emphysema.[14]

Perhaps the most telling of all evidence against cigarettes arises from a simple comparison of annual death rates among smokers and nonsmokers. The famous 1964 U.S. Surgeon

General's report noted that the death rate among men smoking ten to nineteen cigarettes daily is 70 percent higher than that of nonsmokers. For those smoking forty or more daily, the death rate is 120 percent higher. Nearly half the excess —and presumably avoidable—deaths that occur among smokers in a given year result from coronary heart disease, while over one-sixth of them are caused by lung cancer.

Since the major medical indictments of smoking first appeared in the 1950s and early 1960s, further evidence that raises questions about human rights has accumulated. Voluntarily inhaling carbon monoxide and carcinogens is one thing; exhaling them into the air that others are forced to breathe is quite another. In a smoky room or car, nonsmokers inhale tars, nicotine, and carbon monoxide just as smokers do, and both groups register at least temporary changes in their blood. Breathing the exhaust of smokers can thus strain the heart patient who does not smoke. One study conducted in poorly ventilated saloons in Cleveland found that, over the course of an eight-hour shift, bartenders inhaled as many noxious fumes as would those who smoked thirty-six cigarettes in the same amount of time.[15] Once mainly a symbol of behind-the-scenes political bargaining, the "smoke-filled room" could well take on broader connotations as medical research on smoking expands.

The most potentially tragic victims of cigarettes are the infants of mothers who smoke. They are more likely than the babies of nonsmoking mothers to be born underweight, and thus to encounter death or disease at birth or during the initial months of life. In an otherwise supportive environment, the infant is usually well equipped to withstand the impact of maternal smoking. But when other factors that imperil the newborn are present, such as poverty or poor maternal nutrition, heavy smoking by the mother nearly doubles the infant's odds of dying within a month of birth. Moreover, whether or not they are born underweight, the infants of smoking mothers suffer more bronchitis, pneumonia, and other chest infections than other infants do.[16]

Many people have extinguished their last cigarettes after learning of the health consequences of smoking. The proportion of cigarette smokers among the U.S. adult male population has fallen from 53 percent in 1964, the year in which the Surgeon General's report appeared, to 39 percent in 1975. Among U.S. adult women, the proportion of smokers fell from a high of 34 percent in 1966 to 29 percent in 1975. In Great Britain and several other countries, smokers have also shrunk in number. As a second-best response to the perils of smoking, still other new and veteran smokers now buy cigarettes that contain relatively low amounts of tar and nicotine. The figures, then, show a significant, though hardly revolutionary, reversal of smoking trends in some of the more developed countries. They also show that the decline in smoking has been especially marked among the most highly educated people. In the United States, half of all college graduates who have ever smoked regularly have dropped the habit.[17]

The overall downturn in U.S. smoking rates has been marred by a notable exception—one that accounts largely for the slight increase in overall U.S. per capita cigarette consumption since it hit its lowest point in recent history in 1970. Unprecedented numbers of teenage girls and young women now smoke. Urged on by the efforts of the tobacco advertisers to identify smoking with women's liberation, young women are narrowing the historic gap between male and female smoking rates. In fact, in the fifteen-to sixteen-year-old age group, a slightly higher proportion of girls (20 percent) than boys (18 percent) now smokes. Twenty-seven percent of all U.S. teenage girls now smoke regularly and the number is climbing in the United States and many other countries—a trend that a WHO committee has found especially troubling in light of "the clear finding that smoking during pregnancy has adverse effects on the fetus."[18] If, as one familiar cigarette ad patronizingly chants, women "have come a long way," women's equality with men as smokers may lead to nothing more "liberating" than premature death.

Although the percentage of its population that smokes is somewhat smaller than it was a decade ago, the United States retains its longstanding title as the world's premier cigarette-smoking country. Partly because so many Americans smoke, but also because U.S. smokers tend to smoke more cigarettes per day than most other smokers do, about 2,750 cigarettes were smoked in 1974 for every person in the country. Only Japan, with a 1974 per capita consumption of 2,600 cigarettes, came close to the U.S. average; astonishingly enough, 70 percent of all Japanese men smoke, though only 9 percent of Japanese women do. Annual per capita cigarette consumption in Western European countries ranges from 1,000 to over 2,000; average consumption in Mexico is over 700 a year; and per capita consumption in poor African countries like Nigeria and Tanzania is still only a few hundred cigarettes per year.[19]

These national cigarette-consumption averages provide little hint of the present smoking pandemic. While the incidence of cigarette smoking may have peaked in some of the developed Western countries, the practice has entered a dramatic growth phase in most less developed countries. Cigarettes are catching on especially quickly in the cities of the poor countries, the forges of "modernization." A recent Pan American Health Organization survey in eight urban areas of Latin America revealed that an even higher percentage of men in these cities than in U.S. cities smoke: 45 percent. In contrast, 18 percent of the women in these major Latin American cities are smokers.[20] Sensing the limits of sales potential at home, the major cigarette companies are now as

never before aiming their promotional powers at developing-country markets.

Cigarette smoking is not yet a national pastime in most of
Africa and Asia as it is in Latin America—no doubt in part
because average personal incomes in Africa and Asia are
generally much lower than those in Latin America. Ironically, however, just at the time when the smoking habit is
being dropped by record numbers of the best-educated and
better-off people in North America and Western Europe, the
educational and economic elites of the world's poorer countries are leading their countrymen in taking up the practice.
Data from India, Uganda, and elsewhere show that cigarette
smoking is especially popular among university students.[21]
In hand or mouth, the cigarette seems, oddly enough, to
bespeak privilege and knowledge.

Perhaps the chief constraint on cigarette use in poor
countries is money: only the rich can afford more than an
occasional smoke. As incomes in Africa, Asia, and Latin
America rise, both the number of smokers and their smoking
frequency climb as well. Rapid income growth usually affects
smoking rates perceptibly; oil-rich Middle Eastern countries
are providing cigarette merchants with a hot new market. In
Nigeria, lung cancer is still rare, but a medical professor at
Lagos University warns that "lung cancer will emerge with
the affluence generated by our country's oil economy; there
will definitely be more money for cigarettes."[22]

Smoking in poor countries is by no means confined to
urban areas. Tobacco use has long been entrenched in many
rural regions. For example, shredded tobacco for hand-rolled
cigarettes or pipes is a stock item in every Indonesian marketplace. In China, the amount of tobacco grown in backyard
plots for personal consumption probably rivals the output of
the vast state-run tobacco industry. Contemplating the dim
nutritional prospects of the Gurungs, a hill tribe of Nepal,
anthropologist Alan MacFarlane recently wrote that, faced

with a financial pinch, the tribespeople would likely let themselves become "malnourished rather than give up certain 'luxury' goods such as cigarettes."[23]

Who profits from the tobacco business? The long list of those with a financial stake in a booming cigarette trade includes private and governmental tobacco farmers, huge transnational private cigarette companies and state-owned cigarette monopolies, local and national governments that collect tobacco-generated taxes and foreign exchange from tobacco sales, and the thousands of newspapers and magazines that carry cigarette advertisements.

The two leading tobacco-growing countries are China and the United States; India, the Soviet Union, and Brazil come next but far behind. But the world's five major cigarette companies are, in order, the Chinese Government monopoly, the British-American Tobacco Company, the Soviet Government monopoly, the Japanese Government monopoly, and Philip Morris, Inc.[24] Hence three of the top five cigarette producers are public rather than private enterprises.

The nearly unfettered functioning of cigarette companies in capitalist social systems—in which the ethic of "free enterprise" is deeply entrenched, if not always obeyed—is predictable. But the seemingly unchecked power of tobacco interests within the governments of controlled-market economies such as those of China and the Soviet Union is rather puzzling to some observers, particularly since both those governments have so strongly emphasized preventive medicine. While the Soviet Government is at least trying to discourage smoking through public education, the Chinese Government has done nothing to uproot the habit. When hunger and unsanitary living conditions were the overriding health challenges in China, an anticigarette campaign probably would have been a luxury. But now, following China's dramatic

successes in reducing undernutrition and infectious disease,
cigarette-induced ailments are on the increase. Admittedly,
antismoking campaigns would probably have struck the Chinese as hypocritical, since many powerful national leaders—
including the late Chairman Mao—have been heavy smokers. But a U.S. Senate staff member offered a second explanation upon recently returning from a visit to China: the large
tax on cigarette sales "serves as a major source of investment
capital for the central government—a source not easily replaced and therefore not lightly abandoned."[25]

Many governments must view the tobacco trade with
mixed emotions. As they boost cigarette and tobacco taxes
and import duties—often ostensibly to discourage smoking—
governments simultaneously create a major revenue source
that is far easier to justify politically than increases in other
kinds of taxes would be. In many countries, the tax revenue
from tobacco products exceeds the amount received by the
farmers for the original tobacco crop. In the United States in
1974, the federal, state, and local governments took in about
$6 billion in taxes on tobacco products, while the $4 billion
in tobacco taxes received by the British Government in that
year constituted 70 percent of the consumers' expenditures
on cigarettes. Even in Nigeria, where proportionately fewer
smoke, tobacco taxes provided 2.2 percent of all the federal
government's tax income in 1969/70.[26]

Held hostage to the political power of the tobacco and
cigarette producers, or lured by self-interest in the tobacco
business, or both, many governments actively subsidize tobacco production. Dr. Samuel Epstein calculates that the
U.S. Department of Agriculture spends about $50 million
annually on price supports, tobacco research, export promotion, and other programs that support the tobacco industry.
The nation's Agricultural Research Service, Epstein notes,
"assigns more space to research on tobacco than to research
on food distribution. What's more, the A.R.S.'s concern is to

produce a more marketable product, not a safer product."[27]

Governmental double standards are especially flagrant as far as tobacco and cigarette exports are concerned. Foreign exchange is always welcomed by economic planners, and, in this case, the negative health results are someone else's concern. Reading the reports of agricultural economists and officials concerned with tobacco trade, one would never suspect the nature of the commodity they describe. In their insular statistical world, a fall in British cigarette consumption (and hence tobacco imports) is characterized as a "challenge," a swelling of the Middle Eastern cigarette market as an "opportunity."

To help keep Italy's tobacco exports competitive outside the European Community, the EEC provides a subsidy of about ten cents for each pound of tobacco sold. The U.S. Government ended its direct export payments in 1973, and its practice of sharing equally with producers the costs of export promotion in 1975. But the Federal Government still finances trips of tobacco experts to and from the United States, and still finances the U.S. tobacco booths in foreign trade fairs.

Perhaps the oddest and most questionable use of tobacco by the United States has been the inclusion of tobacco in the Public Law 480 "Food for Peace" program of concessional agricultural sales to needy countries. This supposedly humanitarian aid program has been manipulated to meet several goals at once: to get rid of unwanted domestic tobacco surpluses, to introduce foreigners to U.S. tobacco in hopes of nurturing a future commercial market, and to provide economic aid to politically favored governments. The amount of tobacco shipped on easy terms under P.L. 480 has ranged in value from $17 to $35 million a year over the last decade, with the bulk going to areas of "national security" concern such as South Vietnam, Cambodia, and, most recently, Egypt.[28]

Those who design, print, or broadcast cigarette advertisements also benefit from the tobacco business. Far from bringing down the promotional fever a few degrees, the bans on television and radio cigarette advertisements in the United States and in several other countries merely provided a windfall for the print media. Nearly all the $400 million annual advertising budget of the American cigarette companies now falls into the lap of magazines and newspapers. As James Fallows has observed, only a few major U.S. periodicals have distinguished themselves by refusing to partake of this money.[29]

The mainstays of the tobacco business are, of course, the hundreds of millions of tobacco consumers. Social forces encourage people to start and to cling to the smoking habit, but the $85–$100 billion that consumers spend each year on cigarettes is what sustains global cigarette production and trade.

In the ambiguity-plagued universe of environmental-health studies, only rarely does proof of unequivocal links between particular environmental agents and particular diseases emerge. The airtight medical case against cigarettes stands out sharply as an exception. Cigarettes therefore explicitly challenge the capacity of societies to use the conclusions of health research to improve daily life. The selective vision of cigarette-company executives and the smokescreen of cigarette advertising notwithstanding, today's meaningful debate is not over the possibility that cigarettes might be a public hazard. The only question is what to do about a proven hazard.

But getting cigarettes out of the upper hand is no simple task. Pollution from cigarette smoke, unlike impure water or industrial wastes in the air, results primarily from personal decisions. Smoking, overnutrition, dangerous driving, and other forms of self-destruction are all health problems rooted in personal behavior, problems that often leave health officials feeling perplexed and impotent. What are public health officials to do to influence the many informed people who persist in unhealthy behavior despite their knowledge? Draconian interventions into people's lives could probably keep smoking to a minimum but would do so at a steep social price. At the same time, social policy should acknowledge that the individual's decision to smoke does not take place in an ideal world of free, informed choice. Nor is tobacco production solely a free-market response to consumer demand —and the full costs of smoking are by no means borne by tobacco consumers alone.

From infancy onward, people are bombarded constantly with subtle and not-so-subtle enticements to smoke; powerful advertisements that associate cigarettes with sexual success are reinforced by what is probably a far stronger influence—the example set by countless smoking adults. Although teenagers may start smoking out of desire to appear suave and mature, they may keep smoking long after that motive has lost its relevance because they are hooked on nicotine, an addictive drug.[30]

The full social cost of cigarette smoking has never been calculated, but the purchase price of cigarettes, the extra medical expenses incurred by smokers, and the income that smokers sacrifice to unnecessary disease and premature death together constitute only a portion of the total cost. A 1975 report to the Massachusetts Public Health Association estimated that Massachusetts smokers alone cost the general public more than half a billion dollars a year. If no one in the state smoked, fire protection costs would fall by at least $18 million, and fire damage would fall by at least $24 million a year. Medical care provided with public funds or health insurance to treat smoking-induced diseases costs $220 million a year. Production losses in the state totaling $260 million a year result from the working time missed because of smoking-related disease.[31] If the Massachusetts rate holds for the

entire country, American smokers account for some $19 billion in public expenses and production losses.

The cost of cigarettes also includes the many hundreds of millions of dollars in public funds spent around the world each year on research on smoking-related cancer, heart, and respiratory diseases. Moreover, nonsmokers generally pay higher life insurance rates than they would if smokers were not included in the actuarial tables. The health hazard that smokers inflict upon innocent bystanders provides another critical justification for governmental interventions to deter tobacco use.

These various considerations both provide the rationale and suggest some desirable outlines for public policies on smoking. Each country will adopt a program tailored to its unique smoking problems and social values, but certain policies seem appropriate nearly everywhere.[32] In all public places, either smoking bans or special smoking zones must be put into effect. The need to reduce tobacco-related health risks to involuntary smokers surely transcends any individual "right" to smoke in public. Because it involves actions inside the home and family, the question of fetal and infant risks from maternal smoking constitutes a rather more complex and controversial political issue. At the least, however, all girls and pregnant women must be made aware of the potential impact of cigarette smoke on the unborn and on the newborn.

Over the last few years many local and national governments have, in fact, restricted public smoking. Moscow recently banned smoking in the city's restaurants, while smoking in public buildings and transportation has been limited or prohibited in many parts of the United States and Europe. Such laws are often laxly enforced, however. Interestingly, more than half of all current smokers polled in the United States in 1975 agreed that cigarette smoking "should be allowed in fewer places than it is now"—strong evidence that public opinion is progressing faster than public policy in this area.[33]

Governments can weed many contradictions from their present policies by ending all subsidies to tobacco growers and to tobacco and cigarette exporting concerns. Short-term social difficulties caused by such a move—particularly losses of jobs and income by farmers and workers—could be offset in many cases by using the money once devoted to tobacco subsidies to retrain workers and to introduce more beneficial crops, such as vegetables or soybeans, onto tobacco lands. In any case, temporary hardships resulting from, say, an end to tobacco price supports can be weighed meaningfully only in relation to all the direct and indirect social costs of continued widespread smoking.

In the end the only way to solve the smoking problem is to steer young people away from the habit and to help older smokers kick it. The vigorous, systematic use of all possible educational channels, advertising restrictions, health warnings on cigarette packages, tax disincentives, and so on might alter the smoking scene radically.

A different approach to the problem is to press ahead with the search for cigarettes that are lower in tars, carbon monoxide, and other toxic gases. Both the cigarette companies and the U.S. government are now involved in research toward that end. While opinions differ as to whether public funds ought to be diverted from antismoking campaigns into such research, or whether all such expenses ought to be borne by the private companies, safer cigarettes can undoubtedly reduce the health costs of smoking.[34] The two goals, a nonsmoking society and less harmful cigarettes, need not be viewed as contradictory; both can be pursued at once.

In the world's more developed countries, personal behavior has emerged as a dominant influence on health. The relevant personal choices are in turn influenced by the social and political environment in which people live. Governments

cannot and, most would agree, should not try to dictate medi-
cally rational behavior to each individual. But neither should
they encourage self-destructive behavior. As Dr. Daniel
Horn, one of the pioneers in the study of smoking and health,
says, today's challenge is "to identify the means whereby we
can help people—whether children or adults—to develop
the capability of understanding the issues in personal-choice
health behavior, and the capacity to make choices both in
their own self-interest and in the interest of society at
large."[35]

7. Something in the Air,

AT LEAST since humans discovered fire, air pollution has blighted society. Breathing itself alters the composition of the air, but cooking and keeping warm probably generated the first air "pollutants." Manufacturing and mechanized transportation only stepped up a process older than civilization. The nature and degree of air pollution have varied over the millennia, and humans' attitudes toward it have also changed: heightened concern about polluted air has probably contributed more than any other factor to the recent surge of environmentalism.

The campfires of prehistoric people undoubtedly caused noticeable pollution. The smoky air inside caves, tents, or homes, and sometimes around whole villages, irritated the eyes and encouraged lung and heart disorders. (So it often does today in the homes of the half of humanity that cooks with wood or dried dung; under the right meteorological conditions, the smoke of cooking fires fills huge valleys with a haze that looks like modern urban smog.) But with hunger, wild animals, and the weather gods to contend with, few probably felt threatened by smoke, and the health toll of air pollution was most likely negligible. Indeed, fire and smoke meant food, warmth, and kinship.

As populations and cities grew, so the level of pollution caused by wood smoke must have grown. Pollution was not perceived as a problem, however, until coal was substituted for wood in the early Middle Ages. The imprudent depletion of forests in Britain and in parts of Europe gave rise to this historic transformation in environmental thought.[1] As early as 1306, a Proclamation by Edward I banned the burning of "sea-coales"—chunks of coal found along the seashore—by London craftsmen. At least one unlucky lawbreaker was executed on this count.

Further efforts to control pollution by restricting the ever expanding use of coal were made during the reigns of Richard II in the late fourteenth century and of Henry V in the early fifteenth century. The smoke and odors of coal combustion were seen as public nuisances worth doing something about. But the forces of urbanization and industrialization proved more powerful than love of pure air. Two principal products of coal combustion—smoke and soot—continued to plague societies right up to the mid-twentieth century; and others, especially sulfurous compounds, widely threaten health even today.

In 1661, John Evelyn presented to Charles II a treatise entitled "Fumifugium or, the Inconvenience of the Aer, and Smoake of London Dissipated." Three centuries ahead of his time, he attributed a shortened life expectancy, among other evils, to smoke pollution. An environmental radical, he proposed surrounding London with a green belt and moving all coal-burning industries outside the circle. Like much farsighted advice, Evelyn's was ignored until, much later, immediate self-interest and ghastly events brought the truth home.

The Industrial Revolution and its adjunct, urbanization, together led to a drastic escalation in air pollution. Coal warmed homes, drove factories, and later generated electricity for industrial and residential use. As the nascent chemical industry grew, it too spewed strange new ingredients into the air. In the nineteenth and early twentieth centuries, many cities of Europe and the United States were covered with black shrouds of smoke. As leader of the Industrial Revolution, Great Britain also became the foremost air polluter. London became known for its "pea soup" fog—an unnatural phenomenon that provided Dickens with a metaphor for sickness of the spirit and added flavor to Sherlock Holmes mysteries but shortened the lives of Londoners. Someone coined the term "smog" to describe the combination of smoke and fog that frequently enveloped British cities. Industrial centers like Pittsburgh, Pennsylvania, developed an atmosphere so inky that automobile drivers were sometimes forced to use their headlights at midday.

Laden with compounds that—we now know—cause cancer and respiratory ailments, smoky air must have caused much disease and death. Yet the health costs of air pollution in the early industrial era have never been measured. The dramatic fall in mortality from infectious diseases during this period, a consequence of improved sanitation and diets, easily concealed whatever negative health impact dirtier air had. But it took no sophisticated scientific investigations to establish that heavy smoke pollution reduced the quality of life. Many cities, such as St. Louis and Pittsburgh, embarked on highly successful smoke-control programs in the 1930s and 1940s. London followed suit after a particularly severe smog in 1952 precipitated some four thousand premature deaths in the city. In these cities and elsewhere, smoke and soot proved rather easy to control in comparison with other less visible pollutants.

Up to the mid-twentieth century, smoke and sulfurous compounds were synonymous with air pollution. Thus in 1943, when residents of Los Angeles began complaining about a recurrent, irritating light-blue haze, pollution experts visiting from eastern cities blamed the new problem on sulfur dioxide. But even after industrial emissions of sulfur dioxide were slashed following the passage of a state pollution-control law, the haze appeared with growing frequency. Further studies then showed that hydrocarbons in gasoline vapors could, when exposed to sunlight, combine with other pollutants to form new compounds that resembled those in the Los Angeles sky. Hoping for an easy solution, officials set out to halt the escape of vapors from the gasoline storage tanks of the Los Angeles basin's numerous oil refineries. But still the haze persisted. Finally, the residents of Los Angeles, and ultimately people everywhere, had to face the fact that humans had developed a massive new means of polluting the air: the automobile.

With intermittent spells of atmospheric stagnation and geographic conditions that favored the birth of the car culture, Los Angeles introduced the world to photochemical oxidants—concoctions of ozone and various compounds that form when hydrocarbons (mostly the product of imperfect combustion in engines) and nitrogen oxides (produced both by vehicles and electric-power plants) react in the presence of sunlight. The term "smog" was soon applied to the dark cloud that hung over Los Angeles, and this new use of the word spread quickly, all but pushing its original sense into linguistic history. With the example of Los Angeles before them, pollution researchers everywhere began to reassess local problems and, often, to identify photochemical smog in the air they breathed. As automobile use soared, the familiar haze began settling in over city after city—Tokyo, Ankara, Mexico City, Washington, D.C.

For sheer output, the automobile has no peer; it generates close to half the total tonnage of all air pollutants in some countries. The carbon monoxide emitted by cars is the main offender. Carbon monoxide emissions, most of which come from automobiles, weigh about as much as all other major pollutants combined. Auto-generated hydrocarbons, nitrogen oxides, and photochemical oxidants must also be put on the scale when measuring the impact of cars on air quality.

When the suspected health effects of various pollution sources are compared, however, the automobile remains significant but not so towering. Carbon monoxide is dangerous at high concentrations; but, measured over large areas and at all hours, its health impact is probably far less than that of other rarer pollutants. The health toll of photochemical smog has not been established, but available evidence suggests that it is less injurious than the more traditional London-type smog.

Given what is known about their distribution and their harmful effects, sulfur oxides and particulate matter (varying mixtures of soot, ashes, dust, pollen, sulfuric acid mist, asbestos fibers, and so on) apparently foster more disease than auto emissions do. These pollutants derive primarily from what in the parlance of pollution control are called "stationary sources"—electric-power plants, factories, and homes. Sulfur oxides and particulate matter tend to be concentrated most heavily where coal is widely burned and are usually worst in the winter, when extra combustion is needed to provide warmth. Photochemical smog, in contrast, usually thickens in the summertime.

Sulfur oxides and particulate matter, while comprising only a fourth of all emissions in the United States, probably account for over half the health problems caused by air pollution. Automobiles, a committee of the National Academy of Sciences contends, generate only between one-tenth and one-fourth of the health hazard, even though they create half of all the air pollution in the United States. But even this portion of the hazard could add up to some four thousand deaths and four million days of illness each year.[2]

In addition to the major categories of air pollutants, several other hazardous substances circulate in the air of one place or another.[3] Most ubiquitous of the dangerous heavy metals is lead, a common gasoline additive. Airborne nickel, cadmium, beryllium, and mercury are comparatively rare, but they pose threats in some regions. Carcinogenic asbestos fibers are being discovered in urban air all over the world. Finally, traces of radioactive fallout from above-ground nuclear tests have rained upon virtually everyone.

Air pollution was long associated with economic prosperity and urban growth; today, neither association holds completely true. The worst pollution is generally found, as it always has been, in those large urban areas where air circulation is impeded or is naturally slow. Yet air pollution now threatens more than city folk.

A 1974 study of air quality downwind of the New York City area revealed that people living in Massachusetts as far as three hundred kilometers to the northeast of Manhattan are inhaling the metropolitan area's airborne refuse. During the time it takes for photochemical reactions to occur, the city's pollutants drift northward; thus Connecticut residents living more than forty kilometers away breathe ozone concentrations higher than those found in New York City. Similarly, balloonists who left St. Louis in the summer of 1976 found, when their craft landed in an Indiana wheat field 240 kilometers away, that the pollutants had scarcely thinned out at all.[4]

Light enough to ride the winds, air pollution can be an international threat. Acid rains falling on Sweden and Norway and stunting timber and fish production there are primarily attributable to sulfur emissions in the United Kingdom and Western Europe. By raising smokestacks higher to disperse their own pollutants, the British and the Germans are killing trees and fish in Scandinavia. Similarly, Mexican health officials have discovered dangerous quantities of lead in the blood of thousands of children in Ciudad Juarez; the apparent source is a smelter in El Paso, across the border in the United States.[5]

The simple identification of air pollution with prosperity

can be misleading in two ways. First, the most widespread air pollution, which comes from cooking over open fires with wood or dried dung, afflicts mainly the world's poorest half. Second, while introducing power plants, factories, and automobiles to a region does usually raise pollution levels, the attendant prosperity is not necessarily shared equally by those breathing the acrid air. Commonly, the poorest people in a city live in the most polluted areas, breathing emissions generated by the more affluent to serve their own needs.[6]

Air pollution can become a deadly problem in cities where the vast majority of people are extremely poor. Studies conducted in Calcutta, India, reveal that street-level carbon monoxide concentrations at peak hours rival those in New York, Washington, and Los Angeles. In parts of Calcutta, airborne lead concentrations reach levels higher than those in Cincinnati, Philadelphia, and Detroit. The hundreds of thousands who live on Calcutta's sidewalks probably suffer most from the city's air pollution, which seems to result primarily from the general use of aged, poorly tuned vehicles.[7]

Although anyone inhaling badly polluted air intuitively senses the implicit peril, establishing the exact health hazard posed by air pollution is difficult. Disease and death rates reflect so many factors that the impact of one pollutant alone, let alone of several combined, cannot be pinpointed. The global spread of cigarette smoking in particular has rendered the medical detective's job exceedingly complex, since this form of self-pollution spawns many of the same ailments that air emissions do. Furthermore, doctors do not fully understand the biological mechanisms by which most air pollutants cause disease. As a result, much evidence linking chronic air pollution to ill health remains circumstantial and ambiguous, and some have even called air pollution "a cause in search of a disease."

But such a label is no longer justified, if it ever was. Scores of studies over the last few decades have assembled, bit by bit, a powerful medical case against air pollution. Strong evidence now links air pollution of the levels prevailing in many cities to the heightened incidence of a variety of respiratory diseases. Unfortunately, however, the exact health impacts of particular pollutants and combinations, as well as the precise relationships between pollution levels, duration, and disease, remain unknown.

No one questions the dangers of high concentrations of substances such as lead or carbon monoxide. Nor does anyone doubt that unusually high concentrations of sulfur oxides and particulate matter exacerbate the symptoms of chronic respiratory and heart diseases, sometimes making the diseases lethal. Recounts of the more dramatic air pollution emergencies, especially those in the Meuse Valley, Belgium, in 1930 (six thousand ill, sixty dead); Donora, Pennsylvania, in 1948 (six thousand ill, twenty dead); and London in 1952 (tens of thousands ill, four thousand dead) are prominent in the annals of environmental health. In each of these cases, several days of exceptionally filthy air boosted disease and death rates well above normal.

Death-dealing pollution episodes continue to occur from time to time. Documented jumps in the New York City death rate during periods of severe pollution in 1953, 1963, and 1966 each involved hundreds of excess deaths. Investigations of a four-day period of intense pollution in Pittsburgh in November, 1975, suggest that the foul air killed fourteen people— graphic proof that the city's progress in controlling smoke has not hit the jugular of the pollution problem.[8]

Viewing the concept of a "pollution episode" in a subtler light, researchers correlated day-to-day mortality rates with sulfur oxide levels in New York City. They found that the frequency of deaths from all causes rises and falls with pollution regardless of climatic conditions. Similarly, mortality rates in Los Angeles peak and slump along with the level of carbon monoxide concentrations.[9]

As unnerving and senseless as severe pollution episodes are, considered alone they provide no convincing evidence that air pollution *causes* disease. In each of the incidents just noted, those people with pre-existing respiratory or heart conditions accounted for virtually all the extra deaths. Hence, temporarily heightened death rates prove only that extreme pollution intensifies the severity of existing diseases. Furthermore, temporary jumps in mortality do not reveal the impact of inhaling low or moderate levels of air pollution for years or decades on end. Yet, solid evidence shows that chronic air pollution is a health hazard.

Logically, dirty air should affect the lungs. Accordingly, the role of pollutants, especially of sulfur oxides and particulates, in promoting respiratory ailments has received considerable attention. The general category of respiratory diseases includes both acute, short-term afflictions (such as colds, bronchitis, and pneumonia) and chronic ailments (such as asthma, chronic bronchitis, and emphysema, the latter two of which strike mainly older people); it usually excludes lung cancer.

In every country, respiratory diseases engender more illness than do all other diseases combined. The common cold —an infection of the upper respiratory tract—is by far the world's most prevalent disease. Infections of the lower respiratory tract such as bronchitis and pneumonia frequently take lives, especially in poor countries. In rich countries, especially in regions with heavy air pollution, chronic respiratory diseases are significant causes of death, though they rank far below cardiovascular diseases and cancer.

Chronic respiratory diseases, especially chronic bronchitis, take the highest toll in the United Kingdom, where they claim direct responsibility for nearly 6 percent of all deaths. In the United States, they account for over 2 percent of all deaths; in both countries, they contribute to many more deaths as well. Because of their long-standing experience with chronic bronchitis, British doctors are more likely than those elsewhere to recognize its symptoms. But the percentages do not merely reflect diagnostic discrepancies. In 1964, leading British and American researchers who jointly studied respiratory disease mortality in their two countries concluded not only that the difference in overall rates was real, but also that the higher average exposure to sulfur oxides and particulate matter in England probably accounted for the disparity.[10]

In the United States, the number of recorded deaths from chronic bronchitis and emphysema doubled every five years between the late 1940s and late 1960s. Emphysema, which is manifested as an increasingly severe shortness of breath, now torments 1 percent of all adult Americans and kills more than 20,000 a year. Chronic bronchitis afflicts 3 percent of all adults but takes fewer lives, roughly 5,000 annually. Asthma kills about 4,000 Americans a year but afflicts far more—about 4 percent of the general population.[11]

Cigarette smoking almost certainly ranks as the chief cause of chronic respiratory diseases. The soaring incidence of these diseases in the United States has followed, with a time lag, the spread of smoking during this century. Wherever they live, smokers are far more prone than nonsmokers to contract lung diseases. But air pollution clearly pushes up the incidence and severity of both emphysema and chronic bronchitis, and dirty air severely aggravates the symptoms of many kinds of asthma.

The lungs of those dying in St. Louis—a city heavily polluted with sulfur oxides, nitrogen oxides, hydrocarbons, and particulates—have been compared with the lungs of those dying in Winnipeg, Canada—a city of relatively clean air. Emphysema is both more common and more severe in St. Louis than in Winnipeg. In neither city do the lungs of nonsmokers display severe emphysema, suggesting that cigarettes play a dominant causal role. But smoking residents of St. Louis are four times as likely as smokers in Winnipeg to develop severe emphysema. Smoking and air pollution seem to operate synergistically in promoting the disease.[12]

Numerous studies conducted in the United Kingdom and the United States have shown that long-term exposure to sulfur oxides at now-common levels often causes chronic bronchitis. In the early 1970s, health surveys comparing polluted and nonpolluted communities in four regions of the United States were carried out by the Environmental Protection Agency. The overall conclusion was that, while smoking is the largest determinant of bronchitis prevalence, "air pollution itself is a significant and consistent contributing factor."[13]

Studies carried out in the United Kingdom also reveal that smoking habits relate closely to the incidence of chronic bronchitis. But differences in smoking patterns alone cannot explain why the condition prevails more often in urban than in rural areas. A survey of post office workers in London and in three rural areas suggests that "air pollution is the major reason for the excessive frequency or severity of chronic bronchitis in London."[14]

Air pollution not only promotes chronic diseases; it also boosts the frequency with which people, especially children, contract short-term respiratory ailments. People who live in polluted areas fall ill more often with chest infections of all sorts than do people who breathe clean air. Other factors, including poverty and crowding in the home, push up the incidence of these diseases; but urban air pollution has an additional, independent effect on their incidence. Data from Brazil, Mexico, Japan, the Soviet Union, the United States, and the United Kingdom consistently carry this message. In heavily polluted areas of England, for example, infants under the age of two suffer three times as many lower respiratory infections as do babies in England's cleanest areas. Similarly, according to studies conducted in Nigeria, Colombia, and

India, pollution inside the home from the burning of fire-wood also promotes respiratory infections.[15]

Respiratory diseases obviously lead to the loss of school and work days, to discomfort, and sometimes to death. But the evidence that pollution encourages chest diseases in children holds special significance, for falling victim to respiratory diseases repeatedly during childhood may have a lasting effect, contributing to the onset of torturous and often deadly chronic lung diseases later in life.[16] Children growing up in a polluted atmosphere may suffer for it decades later.

Air pollution's contribution to death by coronary heart disease is increasingly recognized. Heart patients account for many of the extra deaths during pollution crises, perhaps partly because labored breathing strains the heart. Another partial explanation may be that carbon monoxide, a major pollutant wherever automobiles are widely used, promotes cardiac deaths; the presence of inhaled carbon monoxide from cigarette smoke or heavy traffic reduces the blood's capacity to provide oxygen to body tissues. Even in moderate concentrations, carbon monoxide apparently taxes the heart.[17]

While cigarettes clearly contribute to most cases, air pollution also seems to abet the modern lung-cancer epidemic. Residents of large U.S. cities are 20–30 percent more likely than those who live in the country or in small towns to develop lung cancer. Although more urban than rural people smoke, this factor does not fully account for the disparity in cancer incidence. Urban nonsmokers are three to four times as likely as rural nonsmokers to develop lung cancer.[18]

Occupational exposures or unidentified aspects of urban life could be promoting lung cancer, but air pollution appears partly responsible for the rural-urban difference. In Los Angeles in the late 1960s, males living in the neighborhoods most polluted by industry suffered 40 percent more lung cancer than did males in other parts of the city. Evidence points to the interaction of pollution and smoking as the most likely explanation.[19]

Industrial emissions often contain known carcinogens. But some constituents of photochemical smog have never even been identified, let alone tested for cancer-causing potential. Particulate matter in the air has been linked statistically with cancers of the stomach and prostate gland; and, some researchers hypothesize, nitrous oxides in the air may combine with other chemical pollutants to form nitrosamines, which are among the most potent known carcinogens. Airborne nitrosamines may help explain why urban dwellers run increased risks of developing lung and other types of cancer.[20]

Lung cancer strikes more often not only in cities, but also near copper, lead, and zinc smelters and refineries. According to the U.S. National Cancer Institute, 17 percent more men and 15 percent more women develop lung cancer in counties containing these industries than in the country as a whole. Arsenic in the air and ground around the plants appears to be the probable cause.[21]

One of the most conspicuous unknowns in the study of air pollution and cancer is the effect of inhaled radioactive particles, which weapons tests have scattered over much of the earth and over the northern hemisphere in particular. Among the various radioactive materials, plutonium appears most dangerous because it disintegrates so slowly. With a half-life of 25,000 years, plutonium released today will remain active for half a million years.

The plutonium threat exemplifies our incapacity to understand, much less control, the environmental demons we create or unleash. No one knows how plutonium causes cancer, whether low doses over time are more or less dangerous than brief exposures to high doses, or what the combined effect of plutonium and cigarette smoke is. Estimates as to how much of the current lung-cancer epidemic is attributa-

ble to nuclear fallout vary widely, and no means for verifying
any of them exist. Dr. John W. Gofman of the University of
California believes that ten thousand lung-cancer deaths in
the northern hemisphere are caused each year by plutonium
pollution; most other leading students of the problem set the
figure much lower, and some feel the proper number is close
to zero.[22]

Since so many agents pollute our lungs, we may never be
able to measure the exact contribution of airborne radiation
to lung and other cancers. But two points are clear. First,
radioactive pollution of the upper atmosphere—from bomb
tests or "peaceful devices" or acts of war—threatens people
the world over. Second, plutonium introduced into the environment by bomb explosions or through leaks from nuclear
power systems concerns both present and future generations. As Dr. John T. Edsall of Harvard University observes,
"more than one Ice Age may come and go" before plutonium
produced today becomes benign.[23]

In the 1970s, some bizarre new potential connections between air pollution and cancer have been discovered. The
stratosphere's layer of ozone molecules, which filters skin-
cancer-promoting ultraviolet waves from sunlight, appears
to be threatened by a variety of human products. Concern
first arose during debates over the desirability of producing
commercial supersonic aircraft. Many scientists feared, and
continue to fear, that the nitrous oxide in the exhaust of a
large fleet of high-flying supersonic planes would deplete the
ozone layer, since this compound reacts with ozone, convert-
ing it into ordinary oxygen. Next, it was postulated that certain compounds called fluorocarbons—widely used as,
among other things, propellants in aerosol cans—may constitute an even greater threat. The fluorocarbons apparently
break down as they reach the upper atmosphere, disintegrat-
ing into chlorine and chlorine compounds that destroy ozone
even more handily than nitrous oxide does. Most recently,

the possible long-term effects on the ozone layer of nitrous oxide pollution from fuel combustion and nitrogen fertilizers have been questioned.

Near the earth's surface, the ozone *surpluses* of photo-chemical smog are a health hazard, whereas far above the earth, ozone *deficiencies* pose a health hazard for life below. Available evidence suggests that a 7 percent de-crease in the stratospheric ozone layer—a decrease that the U.S. National Academy of Sciences sees as plausible over the next century if recent trends continue—might mean a 14 percent increase in the number of skin cancers. Skin cancers already account for half of all malignancies, some 300,000 cases annually, in the United States. Fortu-nately, nearly all cases are simple to cure. But one type of skin cancer, melanoma, can be fatal and accounts for more than 1 percent of all U.S. cancer deaths. A depletion of the ozone layer would also probably cause crop damage and climatic changes, both of which could affect health as well as politics and economics.

By mid-1977, research into stratospheric ozone trends and threats was pressing ahead urgently; and several countries were considering restricting fluorocarbon use, even though the case against these propellants is not closed. Current knowledge of these potential threats has been aptly summa-rized by Dr. Michael McElroy of Harvard University: "There is no doubt that ozone is essential to life, and that atmo-spheric ozone is threatened by certain air pollutants. The problem that remains is to clarify the exact biological conse-quences of serious ozone pollution, and to figure out how to prevent such an environmental disaster."[24] The persistence of problems such as ozone depletion or, to take another ex-ample, the long-term increase in atmospheric carbon dioxide caused by combustion and deforestation on earth, forces upon humanity a new consciousness of the breadth and com-plexity of the natural systems that support all life.

Summarizing the overall health impact of air pollution in the United States, a committee of the National Academy of Sciences has suggested that blame for perhaps 1 percent of all urban illness and death may be laid to dirty air. Other estimates range from below 1 percent to as high as 10 percent. A recent analysis by Lester Lave and Eugene Seskin, for example, concluded that a 50 percent reduction in particulates and sulfates in the air of several American cities would pull down local mortality rates by about 5 percent. Although it sounds small in the abstract, even the 1 percent figure translates as 15,000 extra deaths and 15 million extra days of illness each year. The Academy committee estimates that automobiles may account for up to one-fourth of the total health hazard, with utilities, industries, homes, and other sources accounting for the rest. Any possible toll of radioactive fallout is not considered in these estimates or in most "air pollution" studies.[25]

Air pollution exacts further costs outside the realm of health, wide as that realm is. The pollution damage to agricultural crops, forests, and material goods in the United States alone amounts to a few billion dollars each year. Effluents from nearby industries are damaging India's priceless Taj Mahal, and the Acropolis in Athens is also showing signs of unnatural aging. In Brazil, General Motors had to buy out neighboring industries whose emissions damaged the paint on new automobiles. Copper-smelter emissions in Peru are killing hillside vegetation, sometimes causing spectacular soil erosion.

Also, of course, filthy air exacts a psychic toll of huge dimensions. How can Tokyoites evaluate the near-total loss of their view of the beloved Mt. Fuji? How can people be reimbursed for an assault on the senses by Los Angeles' murky air? One partial measure of the esthetic cost of air pollution is the premium real estate prices that the rich are willing to pay to live in nonpolluted neighborhoods; the poor, of course, must endure the psychological burden of dirty air.

A National Academy of Sciences committee contends that controlling automobile-generated air pollution in the United States could save the nation between 2.5 and 10 billion dollars annually. If the benefits of controlling other pollution sources—whose combined health toll is much higher than that of automobiles—are included, the total possible benefit goes into the tens of billions per year. That a similar amount spent to reduce most kinds of pollution will bring a net social benefit is not in doubt. The problem is to alter the behavior of individuals and corporations in order to realize that social good.

Faced with the world's most intense pollution, the Japanese Government is making a pioneering effort to force those who create environmental health hazards to help shoulder the costs these hazards entail. Under the 1973 Law for the Compensation of Pollution-Related Health Damage, individuals with certain pollution-related diseases are compensated for their medical expenses and lost wages. Upon death, their funeral costs are covered and their survivors receive special benefits. Eighty percent of the compensation funds are paid by the industries that emit the offending pollution. The remainder of the funds come from a tonnage tax on motor vehicles. In 1976, about 44,000 victims of air pollution-related respiratory diseases were compensated under this law, as were a much smaller number of victims of specific pollutants like mercury and cadmium.[26]

Flawless application of such a law is impossible, particularly since so little is known of the precise health effects of various sorts and levels of pollution, and since factors like personal smoking habits cloud the scene. Cancer—the incidence of which is clearly affected by some pollutants—is not covered by the Japanese law at all. The total number of people whose health is being impaired by pollution is undoubtedly many times the number certified for official com-

pensation. More to the point, no amount of money can buy
a new pair of lungs or compensate for the loss of a loved one.

Despite all the difficulties inherent in its application, the
concept underlying Japan's pollution-compensation law may
be worth consideration elsewhere. Any system that makes
polluters pay for the damages they cause has the dual benefit
of encouraging them to cut their pollution and also appor-
tioning more fairly the financial burdens they create. Still,
health taxes should not take the place of stringent pollution-
control standards.

All too visible, air pollution has probably generated more
public interest in environmental quality than has any other
form of environmental destruction. In the countries where it
is most extreme, air pollution is also one of the few environmental problems against which headway is being made in
many countries. This is not to say that air-pollution control
programs have worked perfectly. Progress has been slow,
costly, and troubled by numerous setbacks. Air quality goals
set for 1975 by the U.S. Congress had to be abandoned, and
ambitious plans to reduce auto emission levels by curtailing
city driving have been shelved in response to public resistance. Yet the more developed countries seem committed to
improving air quality substantially over the coming years.

Smoke and soot control has been the area of the most
dramatic improvement. Pittsburgh is no longer the "city of
smoke," and Londoners now enjoy 70 percent more sunshine
in December than they did in 1958. London's sulfur oxide
emissions have also been reduced, but less drastically.[27]

Only within the last decade have most countries begun to
clamp down on major pollution sources other than smoke-
generating activities. Emanating from identifiable stationary
sources, sulfur oxides and many particulates have generally
been easiest to reduce. The broad shift from coal to oil and
natural gas for power generation has in itself reduced sulfur

oxide emissions from utilities. In more developed countries, at least, design changes and pollution-control devices in new automobiles are reducing carbon monoxide and hydrocarbon emissions, but they have been less effective against nitrogen oxides. At the same time the growth in the number of cars on the road tends to offset the gains made by controls on individual vehicles.

Since 1970, after decades of continuous growth, levels of U.S. emissions of all the major pollutants except nitrogen oxides have been falling. In Japan, too, sulfur oxide emissions have recently begun to drop, though photochemical smog continues to worsen.[28] National improvements may, however, conceal the existence of deteriorating local situations. Washington, D.C., for example, experienced its worst smog ever in the summer of 1975, and the Bicentennial summer of 1976 proved even worse.

Where the controls are taking hold, health benefits seem to be appearing already. Carbon monoxide effects on the blood of nonsmoking Chicago residents declined by 18 percent between 1970 and 1974, apparently because the air quality improved.[29]

Beyond the basic resistance of individuals and corporations to spending money and changing lifestyles in order to clean up the air, pollution control efforts have been hampered by inadequate knowledge and technology. In general, we still do not know exactly which pollutants cause what effects. Quantities of a few compounds are commonly measured and correlated with disease patterns, but whether they are the real culprits is seldom known for sure. The technologies of pollution control, such as "scrubbers" that remove the sulfur from coal effluents and catalytic converters that filter automobile emissions, are improving; but they still have drawbacks. Catalytic converters, for example, do not reduce nitrogen oxide emissions substantially, and they may create sulfuric acid mist in auto exhausts. More basic technological gains, such as new methods of combusting coal and new auto engines that produce significantly fewer emissions, are not yet commercially viable.

The global petroleum crisis has further complicated the control picture. American energy officials are urging new utilities to burn plentiful coal rather than relatively clean-burning but scarce oil. As oil and natural gas become more costly and harder to obtain, the increased use of coal for electric power generation and other purposes appears inevitable and poses a major worldwide health challenge.

Although the industrial and automobile pollution in some African, Asian, and Latin American cities is as intense as any in Europe or North America, many cities are just beginning to experience modern air pollution. São Paulo, Mexico City, and others face the same sorts of control challenges that Tokyo and New York do.[30] But many poor countries now have an historically rare opportunity to learn from the development-related mistakes committed by other nations and thus to minimize the negative health consequences that have accompanied rapid economic growth in the West.

Among many in the poor countries, smokestacks and automobiles epitomize prosperity; some people regard warnings about the perils of air pollution as gratuitous attempts to deny the poor the fruits of growth that others already enjoy. But such an attitude belies a fundamental misreading of recent Western economic history. Controlling air pollution need not mean smothering economic progress; instead it can mean redirecting development along lines that entail fewer negative human repercussions. Smokestacks may indeed mean jobs and income; but requiring factories to incorporate available pollution-control equipment or (in some cases) to locate in uninhabited areas need not jeopardize the worker's livelihood.

The association of automobiles with national prosperity is spurious. In Africa, Asia, and Latin America, the private car has become the great social divider between the rich elites and the poor majority, demarcating lives of leisure from lives of drudgery and soaking up funds needed to better the lot of the poor even as it harms the health of all. Many large cities in the West are now fighting (albeit in many cases half-heartedly) to cut the automobile down to size. Its primacy in urban transportation is being challenged by traffic restrictions, improved mass-transit systems, the construction of bicycle paths, and so on. It took OPEC's embargo on oil exports to force Americans to drive less and thus to pollute less, and the improvement was short-lived at that. The question is whether other countries wish to allow themselves to take the same irrational road.

In poor as in rich countries, controlling air pollution involves more than technical issues. Lifestyles, equity, social goals, and, above all, the role of energy in society—how it is obtained and how it is used—must all be considered. Can cities be designed to give all access to affordable transportation while air pollution is minimized? As the era of cheap fossil fuels recedes, can the use of safe, sustainable energy sources—especially the sun—grow until it obviates the need for expanded coal combustion and nuclear reactors? Can general prosperity be achieved in a conservationist, low-pollution society? Could decentralizing population and services hold down pollution levels as it improves the quality of life? Any societies that—either out of scarcity-imposed necessity or out of foresight—find answers to such questions will have much to teach the rest of the world.

8. Who Pays for Production?

THE QUESTION of how to divide up the fruits of labor is a familiar feature of the economic landscape. New questions grow out of the study of occupational health: Who picks up the tab for production? What are its total human costs? As word of occupational diseases and risks spreads, so does the realization that some individuals bear a disproportionate share of the burdens of economic growth. Just as products are seldom distributed equitably, production-related health hazards spare some and ruin others; and those who consume the most are rarely those who pay the heaviest health costs.

That jobs might be hazardous is not a new idea. But until quite recently, both workers and lawmakers failed to grasp the problem's scope. "Occupational health" once usually referred to the attempt by management or unions to limit the number of limbs lost to machinery, eyes damaged by chemical sprays, or lives lost in explosions or mine cave-ins. And, although numerous laws have governed industrial safety since the late nineteenth century, the threat of on-the-job accidents remains real enough. In 1971 in the United States, calculates Nicholas A. Ashford, more than one in forty industrial workers died or suffered a reportable injury on the job. In that year, reported accidents at nonagricultural workplaces in the United States caused more than 14,000 deaths, over 100,000 permanent disabilities, and upwards of two million temporary injuries.[1]

As huge a problem as it is, the "traditional" threat of industrial accidents has begun to pale beside that posed by the occupational diseases that medical detectives are now identifying. The U.S. Public Health Service has estimated that 390,000 new cases of occupational disease appear annually in the United States while up to 100,000 occupational disease-induced deaths occur each year. But because many occupational illnesses develop silently and slowly, the dimensions of occupational disease remain totally unknown. The more the problem is studied, however, the more pervasive it proves to be.[2]

The breadth of the occupational health problem—including both accidents and diseases—boggles the mind.[3] Workers in pre-industrial societies face special health risks just as workers in technologically advanced societies do. Farmers and fishermen in many tropical countries, for example, are especially liable to contract schistosomiasis and other infections spread by waterborne parasites. The grinding physical strain of pedaling bicycle-rickshaws in Kathmandu or of hand-pulling rickshaws in Calcutta may be life-sapping, especially if the driver cannot afford to eat well.

Some work hazards disappear as societies industrialize, but others crop up in their place; and, as economies grow more complex, so do their occupational health problems. For example, workers on mechanized farms suffer high accident rates and risk being poisoned by pesticides or enervated by animalborne diseases and a host of lung afflictions brought on by inhaling the dusts of grains, cotton, tobacco, and other farm products during processing. Textile workers who inhale cotton or flax dusts are susceptible to irreversible lung damage.

No large class of workers faces higher health risks than miners do. In day-to-day mining operations, accidents and large-scale mine disasters occur regularly. But a far greater, though less perceptible, risk is that of disability or death from chronic lung diseases caused by mineral dusts. Ore refiners and processors are often exposed to hazardous fumes and particles, and they die of cancer at higher-than-normal rates.

Industrial workers face a host of perils, old and new. Workers in many factories live with the threat of lead, mercury, or arsenic poisoning. Each year, tens of thousands are robbed of their hearing by the incessant loud noise typical of many factories and construction sites. This same group lives under noise-related stress that may promote cardiovascular and neurological disorders.

The proliferating plastics and petrochemical industries have manufactured a whole new set of hazards. The long-term health effects of many of the hundreds of thousands of chemicals now in industrial use are not known, though Dr. Samuel Epstein estimates that perhaps 10 percent of all cancer deaths in American males have occupational origins.[4] Worker exposures even to known carcinogens often continue as long as the product in question sells. Exposure levels to known cancer-causing agents are usually regulated by governments, but such efforts do not necessarily eliminate health damages because safe exposure levels to carcinogens cannot be determined and may not exist.

Occupational illnesses do not single out blue-collar workers. Those who apply anesthetics daily in hospital operating rooms experience more cancers, more liver and kidney diseases, and more spontaneous abortions than those who don't; they are also more likely than others to bear babies with birth defects. Some job perils seem, in fact, to stem from purely psychological stresses. Air-traffic controllers, a 1973 study showed, suffer a multiplied risk of hypertension as one consequence of their nerve-frazzling job. Job-related stresses, probably in combination with other genetic and lifestyle influences, may also account for an unknown share of the heart attacks that are so frequent in modern societies. Unemployment, of course, has its own hazards: undernutrition in some countries, drinking or overeating in others, and psychic stresses almost everywhere.

Because they directly affect so many people, occupational diseases represent a major public health challenge in their own right. But they carry a broader social significance as well. Like the canaries that coal miners once carried underground to test the air, industrial workers have themselves unwittingly served as a toxic-substance early-warning system. Much of what is known about poisonous or cancer-causing materials has been learned by studying unusual patterns of disease and death among workers—humans, rather than rodents, have been society's guinea pigs. Often, hazards first discovered in workplaces are later found in lower concentrations in the society at large.

Dangerous substances used in workplaces commonly infiltrate the workers' homes and communities. For example, asbestos fibers carried home from factories on clothes and bodies have caused cancer among the families of asbestos workers in at least eleven countries. Simply because they washed their husbands' clothes years earlier, some women are dying of asbestos-induced cancer; merely being in close contact with their fathers has brought some asbestos workers' children the same awful fate. Likewise, recent examinations in the United States have revealed dangerous levels of lead in the blood of lead workers' children, chiefly a consequence of inhaling lead dusts brought home on clothes.[5]

Those working with arsenic in copper, lead, or zinc smelters suffer exceptionally high lung cancer rates. But residents of the U.S. counties in which such smelters are located also get lung cancer more often then normal, apparently because they inhale airborne arsenic emitted by the plants. As National Cancer Institute researchers put it, "the carcinogenic hazard of arsenic may cross plant boundaries into the general community."[6]

The well publicized Kepone scandal of late 1975 provided an especially dramatic example of how pollution can spread beyond the workplace. The incident also brought to light gross failures of corporate and government responsibility. In its sixteen months of operation in Hopewell, Virginia, a company with the ill-suited name of Life Science Products manufactured the pesticide Kepone under incredibly lax safeguards. Toxic dusts filled the air of the small plant (a converted gas station) and drifted into the air, water, and soil of the surrounding countryside. At least seventy Life Science workers (and a few of their family members) began showing odd and terrifying symptoms, including memory loss, speech slurring, eyeball twitching, liver damage, and sterility. Once doctors figured out the cause of the maladies, the plant was closed. But the doctors had no cure to offer the victims, for Kepone poisoning is a new medical phenomenon.

Only after Kepone made news was its presence discovered in waterways around Hopewell and only then was any attempt made to protect the public from this poison. A long stretch of the contaminated James River was closed to fishing, destroying a major industry. Kepone traces were discovered in fish swimming well out in the Chesapeake Bay, into which the James flows, and in some fish as far away as the waters off New York. Then, as the search widened, slight traces of Kepone were found in the breast milk of mothers in several southern states, apparently a legacy of a federal fire-ant eradication program in which a related pesticide, Mirex, was used. (Sunlight and moisture can form Kepone from Mirex.)

So far, all the known Kepone-induced diseases have involved Kepone workers or their families—individuals who have been exposed to large concentrations of the stuff. But the pesticide causes cancer in animals; and the full health consequences, both for Life Science employees and for the

huge numbers of people around the world who have unknowingly ingested minute amounts of Kepone, will not be
known for decades, if ever.[7]

Diseases among workers sometimes provide the first hint
that a material might be unsafe. Asbestos again offers the
most notorious illustration. In the United States alone, at least
one million people now alive have handled asbestos at work.
If past patterns hold, 400,000 of them will die of cancer over
the next several decades—more than twice as many as would
die of cancer among a million average Americans. But virtually everyone in more developed countries has been exposed
to asbestos fibers at some time. Valued for its toughness and
fire resistance, asbestos has been used to insulate buildings
and ships, to line car brakes, and even to filter beers and
wines. Ubiquitous in modern urban environments, asbestos
fibers are present in the streets, in water supplies, and in
offices. While the misfortune of asbestos workers has
prompted efforts to reduce asbestos use, the substance is still
widely employed and the fibers still waft through the air
millions breathe. Undoing an all too typical error, Yale University recently replaced all the ceilings in its ten-story
school of art and architecture because dangerous numbers of
asbestos fibers were flaking off them.[8]

Ancient Greek and Roman writings are shot with references to the diseases peculiar to one or another profession.
The flowering of trade, industry, and metallurgy in the Rennaisance, however, gave rise to the first systematic investigations of occupational health problems. In particular, the rising demand for gold and silver for use in international
exchange and for metals from which to forge firearms and
other products forced the mining industry to expand. As
underground mines grew deeper, they became more dangerous; and miners and metal workers became the first subjects of medical research into diseases of the workplace.

Perhaps the first publication that addressed occupational

hazards and their prevention was a brochure written in Germany in 1472. The pamphlet told goldsmiths how to avoid poisoning by mercury and lead. In 1556, in his treatise on the mining industry, German mineralogist Georgius Agricola included the first known written review of miners' health problems. Agricola observed that some women who lived around the mines of the Carpathian Mountains in Eastern Europe had lost seven successive husbands to mine-related diseases or accidents. According to the late medical historian Henry E. Sigerist, virtually every book on mining after Agricola's contained a chapter on the diseases of miners.[9]

An Italian physician named Bernardino Ramazzini established himself as the doyen of researchers in occupational medicine when he published his witty and thoughtful book, *Diseases of Workers,* in 1700. Ramazzini surveyed the disease threats—and potential measures to prevent them—of dozens of professions. "Many an artisan has looked at his craft as a means to support life and raise a family, but all he has got from it is some deadly disease, with the result that he has departed this life cursing the craft to which he has applied himself," Ramazzini wrote in his book's preface.[10] In calling on his medical colleagues and the law to make workplaces safer for workers, Ramazzini threw down a challenge that has not yet been fully picked up.

For at least two thousand years, some perceptive doctors and individuals have linked specific occupations to specific diseases. Yet somehow those perceptions have never been followed up with the comprehensive research and regulatory efforts needed to keep job-related diseases at bay. To be sure, many doctors, researchers, companies, and workers have contributed valiantly to worker safety and health. And no individual can be blamed for a whole profession's lack of scientific understanding of various disorders. But, at the same time, widespread hazards persist in societies that have the technological and economic wherewithal needed to reduce worker perils radically.

Medicine has advanced markedly since 1866, when a prominent British doctor who had observed the chronic lung diseases suffered by dust-polluted workers recommended that affected individuals "should be induced to preserve the beard on the upper lip, or the moustache, in order to intercept during respiration the mineral, vegetable or animal molecules diffused in the air surrounding them." To this day, however, many production processes are not as safe as they could be. Gaping holes in knowledge about commonly used materials remain; and, more reprehensible, knowledge of hazards is not always carefully marshalled to promote worker safety.[11]

As Dr. Joseph K. Wagoner of the U.S. National Institute for Occupational Safety and Health observes, two centuries have passed since Percival Pott linked coal tars to the scrotum cancer that killed young chimney sweeps in England. Yet thousands of coke-oven workers in steel mills around the world continue to inhale the same deadly substances, and they are dying of lung cancer at ten times the rate of other steel workers. Dr. Irving J. Selikoff tells the sorry tale of American coke-oven workers:

> Starting in 1936 and at intervals thereafter, scientists reported that lung cancer was much more common among men working in plants like this. Yet for the last forty years, a period during which tens of thousands of American men were daily exposed to these cancer chemicals, decades in which they had every right to assume that their workplace was safe, no precautions whatever were taken to prevent their inhalation of these materials. They were not even told of the danger!
>
> . . . steel workers during the 1930s, 1940s, 1950s, and 1960s surely had the right to expect that someone was seeing to it that cancer would not be their fate. *There was no someone.*[12]

Either deliberately or out of negligence, companies and regulators have often kept behind closed doors the research findings and lessons of experience that could save workers'

lives. Many decades back, studies in central Europe revealed
that uranium miners were dying of lung cancer with unusual
frequency. Europeans went on to establish that this risk
could be reduced substantially by installing adequate ventilation in the mines. But, as Ashford writes, the "failure of
public and private decision-makers to utilize this widely disseminated information has exacted a terrible toll among
America's uranium miners." As recently as 1971, thousands of
U.S. uranium miners still worked under conditions that tripled their chances of getting lung cancer. Decades after
Japan and several European countries banned or halted the
use of certain cancer-causing chemicals in the dye industry,
notes Wagoner, "thousands of American workers are still
literally sloshing in them." As many as 50 percent of the
former workers at some plants that produce dye ingredients
have developed bladder cancer.[13]

Either because materials used on the job have never been
tested for potential health hazards, or because industries and
their regulators have ignored test results, nasty "surprises"
about one substance or another appear from time to time.
The discovery of rare liver cancers among dozens of vinyl
chloride workers in 1974 was a harbinger of shocking disclo-
sures to come.

Thousands of chemicals with unknown health effects
have been introduced into workplaces over the last three
decades. Since long lag-times often separate toxic-chemical
exposures from the onset of diseases, tracing the impact of
dangerous chemicals entails extraordinary difficulties. Had
vinyl chloride caused a more common malignancy (such as
lung cancer) than it does, its threat might have gone unrecog-
nized indefinitely. Yet, even in the case of vinyl chloride,
claims Dr. John M. Peters of Harvard University, "well before 1974, there was enough evidence to support the pre-
sumption of a serious occupational hazard."[14]

A county-by-county survey of cancer incidence in the
United States, recently carried out by the National Cancer

Institute, provides strong circumstantial evidence of what most cancer researchers have long suspected. The study indicates that many industrial causes of cancer await identification. In general, cancer rates for both sexes are highest in the most heavily industrialized counties. Comparing the incidences of specific types of cancer with the locations of particular industries, Drs. William J. Blot and Joseph F. Fraumeni, Jr., found excessive lung cancer rates among males living in counties containing paper, chemical, petroleum, and transportation industries. In some cases, the involved industries have not previously been linked to lung cancer. While these correlations may well point to occupational hazards, the researchers write that it will be necessary "to supplement occupational studies with community surveys to determine whether a cancer risk is confined to the workplace or has spread beyond plant boundaries."[15]

The subject of the earliest writings on occupational health, miners have paid with their lives for four centuries to supply societies with coal, minerals, and metals. The effect of coal dust on the lungs has been well known to doctors at least since 1813, when the "black lungs" of autopsied coal miners were described in medical literature. Yet, while countries vary in their concern for miners' welfare, less has been done in most places to control coal-mine dust than could be. In 1974, an editorial in the respected British medical journal *The Lancet* charged that "between the wars, when the introduction of mechanisation without dust control created gross disease on a mass scale, the complacency of experts . . . delayed effective dust suppression for a whole generation." Reviewing the persistence of both pneumoconiosis (black-lung disease) and excess chronic bronchitis among British miners, *The Lancet*—which is not normally given to using inflammatory language—said that "there is overwhelming evidence that coal mining still uses up men and discards them to an exceptional extent."[16]

As recently as the early 1970s, a committee of the U.S.

National Academy of Sciences felt pressed to write that in the United States "the underground control of coal dust must be improved. Proper ventilation technology is available and has been for some time; the high incidence of pneumoconiosis is inexcusable." Recent studies have shown that 8 to 10 percent of U.S. coal miners suffer from black-lung disease. Although the federal government is now trying to bring dust-control in American mines up to the standard that many European countries have long maintained, the health provisions of the 1969 Coal Mine and Safety Act have not been strongly enforced. At the same time, observes the International Labor Organization, coal-mine safety and health conditions in poor countries such as India are generally worse than those in the United States, let alone those in Europe.[17]

Silicosis, another lung disease caused by dusts in mines and quarries, is even more prevalent than black-lung disease. In fact, according to WHO, "of all occupational diseases, silicosis is the major cause of permanent disability and mortality and is the most costly in terms of compensation payment." Although dust-control measures have slashed its toll in many developed countries, silicosis still imperils the health of miners everywhere. Less developed countries have been especially delinquent in suppressing mine dusts. Twenty-three percent of Bolivia's tin miners suffer the chest affliction, as do 14 percent of Colombia's miners.[18]

Agricultural workers rank alongside miners as a group that has paid an especially steep price to satisfy society's needs. Farm workers suffer a disproportionate share of occupational injuries and illnesses. While they constituted only 4.4 percent of the U.S. labor force in 1971, farm workers accounted for about 16 percent of the country's recorded occupational deaths and 9 percent of the recorded injuries; only mine and construction workers have worse recorded safety records. Among farm workers, migrants are usually worst off, since for them the ordinary hazards of the fields are often compounded by unsanitary living conditions, poor nutrition, and extreme poverty.[19]

As if the recorded disease toll of farm work didn't look bad enough, field surveys in all countries reveal far higher agriculture-related disease incidences than official records show. Farm-worker poisoning by pesticides and herbicides is an enormous and generally underestimated problem. Vast numbers of temporary pesticide-induced maladies are either never brought to a doctor's attention, inaccurately diagnosed by doctors, or unreported to public health officials. Many pesticide-caused deaths remain uncounted for the same reasons.

When the California State Department of Public Health carried out a household survey of farm workers in Tulare County, it found that "during 1969, 25 percent of the farm workers had seen a doctor for pesticide-related illness, but official figures put the number at less than 1 percent." The unreported symptoms of pesticide poisoning included nausea, skin and eye irritations, chronic headaches, and sleeplessness. In Nicaragua, where the cotton industry uses pesticides in quantity, 383 deaths and over 3,000 poisonings during the 1969–70 crop year followed exposures to pesticides, according to a report by the U.N. Food and Agriculture Organization. No one can say what the actual health toll of pesticides is in Nicaragua or anywhere else. However, WHO reports that surveys among pesticide sprayers in a number of countries revealed "up to 40 percent of workers with symptoms of poisoning during the spraying period."[20]

Pesticides kill insects by design, and poisonings among some people who apply or work amid them is part of an almost inevitable pattern. But chemicals are often used recklessly, driving the "accident" toll skyward. Pesticides are frequently overused, applied with improper equipment, or used in unnecessarily dangerous combinations. Workers are often sent onto freshly sprayed fields before the greatest danger has subsided; sometimes they are inadvertently doused by airborne sprayers. While such abuses occur wherever pesticides are used, they are particularly common in less developed countries, where farmers and laborers have less education and less experience with modern chemicals than European or North American farmers have. Sometimes the safety warnings and instructions on imported pesticide packages are not even translated into local languages.

Intensifying their occupational hazard still more, farm workers in poor countries are sometimes exposed to pesticides whose use has been banned or carefully restricted in countries with higher testing standards and better chemical-use controls. American and European companies have shown no reluctance to promote abroad pesticides banned in their home countries; and, moreover, their marketing efforts are not always accompanied by candid information about the known or suspected dangers of the products they are peddling.

The pesticide Phosvel, for example, was (until recently) produced in Texas but had never been cleared for U.S. use when, in 1976, severe neurological damage to at least a dozen Texas workers involved in its production became known. Meanwhile, according to Kevin P. Shea of *Environment* magazine, the Velsicol Chemical Corporation (Phosvel's manufacturer) had aggressively marketed the pesticide abroad for use on grain and vegetable crops. Velsicol's advertising brochure in Colombia touted the chemical's safety long after its neurological threat had been scientifically established. In Egypt, which like Indonesia and South Vietnam received the pesticide through the U.S. foreign aid program, Phosvel is believed to have poisoned 65 farm workers, one fatally, in 1975. It also killed several hundred water buffalo there in 1971.[21]

As is the case with so many occupational health threats, the farm workers' pesticide problem is but one part of a

community-wide (in this case, a worldwide) problem. Pesti-
cide-contaminated food is common fare, especially in less
developed countries that lack good inspection systems, and
mass poisonings of consumers are far from rare in Africa,
Asia, and Latin America.[22] "Allowable" traces of a variety of
pesticides grace the food supplies and inhabit the bodies of
virtually everyone in Europe and North America and many
poor countries too. No health consequences related to
chronic, low-level pesticide consumption have yet been de-
tected; cancer researchers are keeping their fingers crossed.

Finally, of course, the specter of irreparable harm to the
complex webs of nature by toxic chemicals has not faded
away since Rachel Carson publicized it in 1962. Already, a
life-threatening ecological side effect of heavy pesticide use
in Central American agriculture has appeared: the evolution
of malaria-transmitting mosquitoes that are resistant to a
wide variety of low-cost pesticides. Malaria-control programs, which rely on the spraying of houses with inexpensive
pesticides, have been severely undermined, and in El Salvador the number of malaria cases jumped from 33,000 in 1973
to 66,000 in 1974.[23]

Within the last decade or so, occupational health has become an issue to more and more scientists, workers, and
governments. The occupational origins of some cancers and
lung afflictions have become more widely understood. The
international communication of relevant medical findings
has escalated. Labor unions in some countries have begun to
show a serious interest in long-term disease threats, as well
as in traditional job safety, and workers are challenging the
historic managerial monopoly on job-related health information. A few countries, particularly some in Scandinavia and
Eastern Europe, have led the industrial world in efforts to
protect workers' health by imposing safeguards within industries and by educating workers about health hazards.[24] Since

the 1970 passage of the Occupational Health and Safety Act, the United States has also moved haltingly toward a more systematic approach to the problem. But, in all countries, much remains to be done.

All indications are that a multitude of occupational influences on disease, especially those that promote cancer, have defied detection. And even known threats are not always being attacked head on. Corporation executives and owners, and often the workers themselves, weigh immediate gains against the uncertain prospect that diseases might develop decades later. In the end, balancing the benefits of producing a particular product against the long-term, imprecise health risks that production entails is as much a matter of social judgment as of economic analysis.

Laboratory experiments and studies of workers' death rates have led to the identification of a growing number of slow-acting disease agents. To date, however, this critical information has not been fully exploited to save lives. Sheldon W. Samuels, health director of the A.F.L.–C.I.O. Industrial Union Division, observes that tens of millions of current and former workers face a verifiably high cancer risk by virtue of their on-the-job exposures to carcinogens. "But even when a high-risk group has been epidemiologically defined," he writes, "we do not notify them, extend surveillance, provide known therapies, or even attempt to expand our abilities to intervene through early diagnosis or treatment of preclinical and clinical disease."[25] Concerted efforts to locate and to provide medical advice to workers who have been exposed to delayed-fuse carcinogens over the last four decades could possibly prevent many premature deaths. But the worldwide task is so huge and fragmented that desultory efforts by a few companies, unions, or researchers will not do.

Meanwhile, in the words of Dr. Selikoff, "seeds are being planted now for the diseases of twenty or thirty years hence."[26] Identifying and controlling hazardous substances before their presence is revealed by epidemics among workers is one of today's most complex and expensive challenges. Laws such as the 1976 U.S. Toxic Substances Control Act, under which pre-use screening of materials will be attempted, and initiatives such as the international registry of toxic chemicals being organized by the United Nations Environment Program are starting points—but no more.

In many African, Asian, and Latin American countries, heavy industries are still few in number and most agriculture has not yet been "chemicalized." The greatest "occupational" problems in such nations cannot be separated from the basic nutritional and sanitational deficiencies that steal years from the lives of the poor majorities. But in virtually every less developed country, small-scale industries are widespread and—whether built by multinational companies, national governments, or local investors—large industrial enterprises are springing up too. Unfortunately, as WHO officials recently said of occupational health with measured understatement, "in developing countries at an early stage of industrialization the significance of preventive action in this field has not always been fully realized."[27]

Many less developed countries have tended to adopt—on paper, at least—the worker-exposure standards recommended by the United States or by WHO. These standards may not, however, be stringent enough to protect some of those in low-income countries who work with dangerous dusts, metals, and chemicals. Analyzing workers' health experiences in several Egyptian industries, Dr. Madbuli Noweir found that serious problems can erupt in people who have been exposed to hazardous substances at levels below those normally accepted in developed countries. He argues that factors outside the workplace, such as the chronic burden of parasitic diseases, poor nutrition, the tropical climate, and various other cultural or environmental influences may increase the susceptibility of many workers in poor countries to harm from toxic substances.[28]

As it does everywhere, worker health competes with

other priorities in poor countries—in particular with the perceived urgency of nurturing economic growth. Moreover, a general shortage of scientists able to monitor and regulate the complex hazards of modern industries hampers those efforts that developing-country governments do make to protect worker health. Thus, in practice, reasonable job-health standards are imposed and enforced far less often in poor than in more developed countries.

The World Health Organization has addressed the special and long neglected health challenge posed by small-scale industries in both rich and poor countries. As WHO observes, two-thirds of all the world's industrial and mine workers are employed by firms that each employ fewer than a hundred workers—firms like a flax-processing facility in Egypt, a scrap-lead smelter in Nigeria, a grain-milling plant in Burma, or a family-owned coal mine in the United States. Often little more than back-yard businesses, small industries rarely provide medical services, and their managers are much less likely than those of large enterprises to keep abreast of advances in occupational-health research and technologies. "Workers in these small industries may well be called the 'forgotten masses,'" writes Dr. M. A. El Batawi of WHO, "for their health problems are rarely of concern to health planners and they receive only marginal attention from labor administrations. Yet, in many countries, such industries form the economic backbone of the community."[29]

The occupational disease problems that afflict women constitute another health category that both rich and poor nations have neglected.[30] While women constitute anywhere from 20 to 50 percent of national workforces around the world, all but a small fraction of occupational medical studies have involved male subjects, and little is known about the differences, if any, in the effects some toxic substances might have on men and women, respectively. A half century back, well publicized abuses of women (and children) in unsafe workplaces spawned laws designed to protect the "weaker" sex. While some such laws eliminated conditions hazardous for anyone, others have given rise to unnecessary discrimination based on incorrect notions about women's physical abilities. Today, however, vexatious new questions about women's occupational health are being raised as more and more women risk exposure and as our medical understanding of toxic substances grows.

The potential for fetal exposures to dangerous substances or radiation is especially troublesome. In the United States alone, at least one million women of childbearing age are exposed on the job to chemicals and metals that might cause birth defects, cancer, miscarriages, or, possibly, behavioral problems. While the developing fetus is probably far more sensitive than an adult to hazardous agents, sufficient knowledge on which to base allowable exposure standards for pregnant women is not available (and some materials may not be safe at any level of exposure). Given the uncertainties, the current trend in some industries is to bar all fertile women categorically from jobs that entail a chance of fetal damage. Women's-rights advocates charge that such wholesale discrimination is illegal and that all women of childbearing age should not be regarded as potentially pregnant. Yet it is true that many women do not realize that they are pregnant for many weeks after conception, during which time irreversible fetal damage could occur.

Increasingly, women are moving into industrial jobs traditionally held by males; and some factories and shops traditionally employ mainly female workers. In both cases, women have the same needs as men—for close medical attention to potential hazards, open access to information about hazards, and for all possible safeguards. Recent research has also suggested that some industrial influences on males' reproductive organs can cause birth defects in the children they father. Clearly, reducing toxic exposures on the job will at once help protect men, women, and their unborn children. Nevertheless, some risk will probably always plague certain jobs, and the need to protect the unborn will continue to pose difficult legal, ethical, and social questions.

Minimizing occupational health hazards is one aspect of economic life that requires strong governmental involvement. The imperative of profits usually conflicts, in the short term at least, with the imperative of worker protection, which costs money. Unless all producers of a given product are forced to comply with strong national standards, competitive economic advantages may flow to the producers that are the least responsive to workers' health needs. For the same reason, minimal international occupational health standards are needed. In an era when corporations will locate production facilities anywhere on the globe that markets and profits are to be found, inadequate health and pollution standards in one country may well seem attractive to investors. But accepting such a trend is tantamount to asserting that a human life is worth less in one country than in another. At present, no authority even keeps systematic track of the worldwide location and movement of hazardous industries, let alone of the health safeguards they adopt.[31]

Those working for cleaner and safer natural environments often ruffle workers, who fear losing their jobs when strict pollution controls are demanded of factories or when construction projects are deemed environmentally unsound and scrapped. As ecologist Barry Commoner observes, however, beneath "their superficial conflict there are deep and powerful reasons for a community of interest between labor and environmentalists."[32] Health hazards in workplaces, like overall environmental degradation, represent production costs that have seldom been counted, let alone billed to those responsible for them. Interjecting both worker and community health considerations more fully into economic decisions will promote better worker protection. It will also insure that, when prevention fails, workers will be more justly compensated for their unwitting sacrifices. Those outside the factories and the farms stand to gain, too, since much deadly pollution begins in workplaces and can be prevented there only.

9. Of Snails and Men

WHEN THE PHARAOH'S daughter rescued Moses from his bulrush basket along the Nile, she was risking more than her father's political disapproval. In the river reeds with the little Hebrew refugee may well have lurked snails bearing schistosomiasis—a strange parasitic disease that has plagued Egypt for millennia and is now spreading in dozens of countries by the careless hands of humans.[1]

In the course of its extraordinary life cycle, the schistosomiasis parasite must spend some time in the human body, some time in water, and some time in certain snails. Thus, the reservoirs and irrigation canals that turn lifeless lands into hospitable human habitats create ideal environments for the parasite-infested snails. Faced with a constantly mounting need for food and hydroelectric power, but short on the resources or the will to control schistosomiasis, governments build new dams and irrigation systems knowing full well that the disease will spread. Already afflicting some 200 million people in at least seventy-one countries, schistosomiasis invades ever more lives each year.

Schistosomiasis primarily strikes the rural poor—one reason why so little has been done to halt its spread, to develop effective cures, or even to document its prevalence. Unlike malaria, to which tremendous attention and resources have been devoted, schistosomiasis poses no threat to the affluent urbanite. Only those who frequent infected canal or lake waters are likely to pick up the blood-fluke, and only where sanitation is poor can the infection persist, since the fluke cannot reproduce unless it is returned to snail-infested water via human body wastes.

Egypt occupies a special place in the history of schistosomiasis. Papyrus documents from four thousand years ago provide the earliest written record of the disease's existence, and some ancient mummies still contain calcified parasite eggs. When Napoleon's troops invaded the Nile delta in 1799, they were invaded in turn by the schistosomiasis parasite. Upon seeing one consequence of the infection among Egyptians—blood in their urine—Napoleon is said to have called Egypt "the land of menstruating men." In Cairo in 1851, Theodor Bilharz first discovered a species of the blood-fluke that causes schistosomiasis and lent his name to the disease, which many still know as bilharzia. Early in this century, as the prevalence of schistosomiasis in the Nile delta grew along with the irrigation system, Egypt became the first country to institute medical treatment and snail-control programs. But over the last two decades, as Egypt poured resources into the construction of the Aswan High Dam, the country's attack on schistosomiasis was not commensurate. Along with year-round irrigation, the dam has brought schistosomiasis to several million people in Upper Egypt. Perhaps two-fifths of Egypt's forty million people now harbor the parasite—a public health burden of staggering proportions.

Though Egyptian scribes first wrote of schistosomiasis, the disease may have originally evolved to the south, somewhere above the headwaters of the Nile River in Eastern Africa.[2] The earliest human-like creatures, most paleontologists believe, emerged in this area. Here, long ago, some of the snail species that host the schistosomiasis parasite may have first developed too. Humanity shared its cradle with the unlikeliest of bedfellows, and the peculiar relationship that links the lives of humans, snails, and blood-flukes was born.

Travelers in a recordless age probably carried schistosomiasis down the Nile into Egypt, from whence it spread to North Africa and the Middle East. Through the centuries, schistosomiasis was gradually carried by migrants and traders to suitable natural habitats throughout the African continent: slow-moving rivers, lakes, and ponds. It may not have reached some parts of Africa until the present century. Ironically, modern-day irrigation developments in Upper Egypt and the Sudan are spiriting the disease back upriver toward its ancient home, allowing the snails and parasites to get a foothold where they once had little chance of surviving.

The construction of countless small-scale irrigation projects as well as of several large dams throughout Africa has afforded schistosomiasis an unprecedented prosperity and prevalence. Every major man-made lake on the continent harbors the flukes, and some variety of the disease now blights every African country except Lesotho. Because of their role in spreading schistosomiasis, many of Africa's major water developments in this century—including Lake Nasser in Egypt, Lake Volta in Ghana, and recent flood-rice projects in West Africa—have been called public-health disasters. Yet, in Africa and elsewhere, more such "seas of troubles" are being created every year.[3]

Schistosomiasis traveled to the Americas in the bodies of slaves during the sixteenth, seventeenth, and eighteenth centuries; almost retributively, the parasite *Schistosoma mansoni* (which invades the intestinal veins) established itself in Brazil, Surinam, Venezuela, and several Caribbean islands. Schistosomiasis failed to sweep across the rest of the New World only because snails of the right sort were not to be found there, which also explains the failure of the urinary type of the fluke *(Schistosoma haematobium),* which is the most prevalent type in Africa and the Middle East, to sustain itself anywhere in the Americas. Infected people, of course, may still take the parasite out of its element, where it cannot reproduce. About 10 percent of the hundreds of thousands of Puerto Ricans who have migrated to New York City have brought the infection north with them. But the presence of sewage systems and the absence of snails prevent schistosomiasis from spreading from person to person in New York, and the blood-flukes inhabiting infected New Yorkers will die off gradually over a five- to thirty-year period.

A third variety of schistosomiasis (an intestinal type caused by *Schistosoma japonicum*) is found only in East and Southeast Asia, and is far more harmful and far more resistant to available treatments than the other two major varieties are. This fierce strain is entrenched to varying degrees in China, Japan, the Philippines, Thailand, Laos, Cambodia, and the Indonesian island of Sulawesi. The possibility that susceptible snails might further invade Southeast Asia's vast irrigation systems, and the likelihood that new river-basin developments such as those contemplated for the Mekong River will proliferate schistosomiasis, are the stuff of which the nightmares of the region's health officials are made.

China, like Egypt, holds a prominent spot in the annals of schistosomiasis. During the first half of this century the most virulent form of the disease afflicted more than ten million Chinese and probably took a greater human toll than it has in any country before or since. Whole villages faced constant misery and even depopulation as the blood-fluke caused liver, spleen, and intestinal problems and early death. Since 1950, however, China has stood out among the handful of countries—also including Israel, Japan, Venezuela, and the territory of Puerto Rico—that have made dramatic inroads against the disease. Chairman Mao was so moved by the progress against schistosomiasis in one region that he wrote a poem about it called "Farewell to the God of Plague."

Among the earth's less developed regions, only the Indian subcontinent, upon which one-fifth of all humanity lives, is

not plagued by schistosomiasis. Mysteriously, urinary schistosomiasis does persist in one village in the Western Indian
state of Maharashtra. But aside from isolated individual cases
discovered from time to time, the subcontinent is otherwise
free of the parasite.

A review of the schistosomiasis parasite's extraordinary
life cycle suggests both the difficulties and the possible means
of eradicating the infection. Few creatures lead such seemingly vulnerable lives. In growing from egg to maturity the
flukes must travel what Dr. Kenneth Warren has aptly
dubbed a "precarious odyssey," relying on the unearned hos-
pitality of two different animal species and on a great deal of
luck for survival. Yet behind the hazardous existence facing
any one of the parasites is a life cycle that all but guarantees
that the species will flourish where appropriate environmental conditions prevail. Adapted to take advantage of the most
basic of human habits and inclinations, the parasites have
time and again revealed exceptional tenacity in the face of
efforts to stamp them out.[4]

The adult flukes inhabit the blood vessels of either the
intestines or the bladder of their human hosts, depending on
the particular species. Each female lays hundreds or, in the
case of the East Asian variety, thousands of eggs per day.
Many of the eggs remain within the host's body, but others
work their way into the bladder or intestines and then exit
with urine or feces. Depending on the severity and type of
their infections, people may excrete anywhere from 100 to
500,000 eggs each day.

If an egg soon reaches fresh water, it hatches and a tiny
larva called a miracidium that swims at about two millime-
ters a second emerges. The miracidium's swim is a desperate
one, for it must find an appropriate snail host within twenty-
four hours or die. The snails evidently exude "perfumes" that
attract the swimming larvae, but still the vast majority perish
before finding a suitable host.

A larva that successfully finds and enters a snail undergoes a remarkable metamorphosis inside the snail's body. It transforms into a sac-like creature that gives birth to hundreds of thousands of juvenile flukes called cercariae. Sometimes killing the snails, this extraordinary, asexual multiplication process takes three to four weeks, after which the fork-tailed cercariae, now slightly less than one millimeter long, take to the water. Outside the snail their survival odds are poor; they have at most two days to find human beings (or, in some cases, certain other mammals) who will, if all goes well for the flukes, provide homes for years thereafter.

Once in contact with human skin the cercariae waste no time, usually worming through the outer layer within minutes. While doing so they undergo yet another profound transformation, dropping off their tails and assuming a worm-like appearance as they forsake fresh water for the salty medium of blood. Within a day or two, the worms burrow through the subcutaneous tissue and into blood vessels, in which they ride to the heart and then the lungs. Pausing there to mature, they then float or burrow to the liver.

While in the liver, the wormlike creatures finally mature into adult, sexually differentiated schistosomes. At this stage, each female worm enters the cleft in a male's body to mate, a position the pair holds for life. Finally, pairs move together to their ultimate destination—the veins of the bladder for *S. haematobium,* the veins of the large intestine for *S. mansoni,* and the veins of the small intestine for *S. japonicum.* So ensconced, the paired schistosomes begin producing eggs, beginning the life cycle anew.

The parasites seldom kill their human hosts outright. (If they did, they probably would have become extinct long ago, for the constant return of huge numbers of eggs into water, which is essential for species survival, would end.) But people who carry large numbers of flukes experience a variety of internal complications, an impairment of their overall physical well-being, and in many cases a shortened life span.

The implications of light infections for the health of individuals, and of widely prevalent infections on community life expectancy, disease rates, and economic productivity have not been established. Why some infected individuals become severely ill while others establish a seemingly harmless relationship with the parasite is another mystery, though recent studies suggest that the number of flukes inhabiting the individual may be the critical variable.

The parasite's initial skin penetration may cause a prickly sensation and, weeks later, when the schistosome pairs begin producing eggs, some people with heavy infections experience a temporary severe fever, weakness and malaise, and other symptoms. Following these stages, many victims show no symptoms for years except telltale blood in their urine or intermittent, often bloody diarrhea.

But whether or not the parasite declares its presence, a heavy schistosomiasis infection may cause irreversible damage that, over time, kills the human host. Less the flukes themselves than their eggs, many millions of which may eventually be deposited in various organs, are at fault. The eggs provoke an intense immunological reaction that destroys and scars tissues and spurs the formation of new fibrous tissue that may restrict the flow of urine through the bladder and ureters, or of blood through the liver. If unendurable pressures build on the kidneys, they may be destroyed; similarly, the abdominal blood vessels around the liver may eventually burst. When heavily infected, even those still in their teens sometimes die from such urinary or liver complications. Urinary schistosomiasis also seems to promote bladder cancer. In Egypt and some other African regions, a fifth of all cancers (and more than a third of all cancers in males) involve the bladder, a fraction vastly higher than exists elsewhere. Ocasionally, the parasite's eggs enter and damage the lungs or central nervous system as well.[5]

The dearth of reliable statistics on the public health impact of schistosomiasis impedes control of the disease. Without hard data on its costs, those concerned about schistosomiasis cannot compete for scarce public resources against those championing causes involving, for example, new electric-power capacity or increased food production. Moreover, the health impacts of chronic, largely invisible diseases are nearly always underestimated—witness the modern epidemic of high blood pressure among the affluent as well as that of schistosomiasis among the poor. Mortality data record fatal crises—the heart attacks and the kidney failures and the bladder cancers—rather than the underlying debilities that make the crises inevitable.

Like most diseases of the poor, schistosomiasis has not received the attention its worldwide significance merits. The annual global expenditure on schistosomiasis research in the mid-seventies was about $8 million, less than a hundredth of the world's cancer research budget. This disparity helps to explain why no completely satisfactory treatment has yet been developed.

Several drugs that can usually kill most of the flukes inhabiting infected individuals are now available. But none works on all people or all species of the parasite, and all pose serious risks for some users. Hycanthone and niridazole, two newer and generally effective drugs with fewer serious side effects than older drugs entail, have shown signs of possible carcinogenic or mutagenic qualities in some animal tests. Yet, after stacking up the known benefits against the risks involved, the World Health Organization and most doctors in the field contend that these drugs ought to be used until their betters are available.[6] As one doctor working in Egypt puts it, "Schistosomiasis not only debilitates and sometimes kills people, but also promotes cancer. We have a drug that can usually cure the disease, but which some animal studies suggest is possibly carcinogenic itself. Under the circumstances, using the drug is certainly the lesser of two evils."

Still, neither doctors nor patients can relish making this sort of choice. Safer, more effective curative drugs or, better yet, a vaccine that confers immunity to infection, are what public health officials throughout the developing world hope to find.

Axiomatically, preventing schistosomiasis altogether is cheaper and safer in the long run than supplying the sick with even the most miraculous drugs. It is in the struggle to halt the constant infection and reinfection of populations that an understanding of the parasite's life cycle becomes so important. If any stage in this cycle can be disrupted through ecological manipulations, then the parasite will be unable to reproduce.

So far in this century, most blows against schistosomiasis have had one point in the cycle as their target—that involving the snails—and have been dealt by one weapon—chemical molluscicides.[7] Control programs are usually aimed at killing the snails in a given area so that newly hatched schistosome larvae will die before locating a snail host. Most have relied so heavily on snail-killing chemicals, not so much because snails are the weak link in the parasitic cycle, but because molluscicides are the most easily managed technological response to the disease. Unlike many other possible control measures, the use of molluscicides does not require large numbers of people to change their habits. Nor does it require planners and engineers to alter their priorities and methods. With molluscicides, a small group of technicians acting alone has a fighting chance of subduing schistosomiasis.

Chemical snail-control programs have worked effectively in several regions, but they have inherent limitations. Hardy and mobile snails that have persevered over many millennia are simply not easily eradicated. Even when most of the snails in an area are wiped out, the survivors can engineer a species recovery, and other snails can be washed into the control area or brought in accidentally by animals or travelers. If even a few people continue to pass eggs into the water, the parasite will reestablish itself after the temporary setback. Hence, once is not enough. Chemical eradication of snails must be an ongoing process, and its high costs must be borne annually unless somehow schistosomiasis is completely extinguished over a large area—an unrealistic prospect at present in most afflicted countries.

Even if molluscicides were not expensive, their ultimate ecological impact would have to be taken into account. As agriculture's experience with pesticides has proven, no chemical's effects can be absolutely controlled. Some molluscicides kill fish as well as infected snails. Benign snail species and other organisms that compete with or feed upon the dangerous snails can also be wiped out by the molluscicide, partially undermining the control effort. The long-term impact of chemical molluscicides on wildlife and people is unknown. Fortunately, the most widely used molluscicide degrades rapidly once in water. But the ecological impact of continuing molluscicide applications over large areas has not yet been adequately studied.[8]

Assessing the threat of schistosomiasis and the effectiveness of chemical snail-control, few control experts rule out molluscicides categorically. But awareness is rising that various nonchemical means of snail control, including both biological and engineering measures, are potentially useful weapons against unwelcome snails.[9] For example, fish and snail species that prey upon the target snails can be introduced into infected zones. Or, irrigation systems can be designed and maintained to frustrate snail life. Nonchemical snail-control measures like these have inspired comparatively little research, and their potential use has often been overlooked. As the United Nations Environment Program has stressed, the tremendous emphasis on chemical means of controlling snails has been at the expense of much-needed attention to other pest-control methods.

In many regions, nonchemical methods of snail control

may prove to be cheaper than molluscicides as well as less threatening to the environment. In parts of Puerto Rico, for example, noninfective snails that squeezed out the dangerous species entirely were introduced at an annual cost of only $0.11 per hundred cubic meters of water treated. Chemical molluscicide programs in Puerto Rico cost $7.50 for each comparable unit of water cleared of snails—sixty-eight times more than the cost of pitting snail against snail.[10]

Where human labor is abundant and well organized, snails can sometimes be eradicated by direct physical means. Together with mass drug therapy and the careful collection and treatment of human wastes, the mobilization of millions of people to kill snails has been a key contributor to China's progress against schistosomiasis. The canals in infected areas are drained, and then the snail-infested mud is dug out and buried in dry land, a practice that is sufficient to kill the snail species prevalent in China. (Some types elsewhere can live for months buried in dry ground.) Following concentrated campaigns of this type, snail-spotters periodically cruise the waterways in canoes, removing with chopsticks any snails they find.[11]

Disease-transmitting snails have suffered the brunt of humanity's attacks on schistosomiasis. But humans, not snails, are the primary hosts and carriers of the parasite. Thus, blocking the cyclical return of eggs from people to water will defeat the disease. Curing infected individuals by using drugs to kill the flukes they carry, for example, can halt the excretion of eggs. But, apart from any medical complications it might entail, mass drug therapy is beyond the financial and organizational means of many afflicted countries—some of which provide rural people with little modern medical care of any sort.

The ideal way to deter transmission of the infection would be to provide people in schistosomiasis-prone areas with reasonably pure water supplies and adequate sanitary facilities

—and then to make sure they use them. Building faucets and latrines for the majority of rural people, who still lack these basic amenities, will carry a stiff price. But, unlike costly molluscicides and drugs, such construction provides a hedge against other social and physical ills too. Pure water and sanitary facilities will cut the crippling burden of infectious disease borne by the rural poor of Africa, Asia, and Latin America. In addition, raw human sewage, a potentially deadly pollutant, can with proper treatment become a valuable resource. Transformed in bio-gas plants or other conversion facilities, sewage can be rehabilitated into usable energy and rich fertilizer even as the schistosomiasis eggs it contains are destroyed. Here again, the Chinese have already proven the practicality of such an alchemical approach, in which a menace is transformed into an asset.

Yet sanitation facilities alone probably cannot flush schistosomiasis from a typical infected region. Safe water and latrines are not completely effective against schistosomiasis unless they are used all the time by all the people. And the universal use of sanitary facilities by rural people has repeatedly proven to be only the pipedream of public health officials. Teenage boys, who generally have the highest infection rates of any age group, are bound to swim in canals or lakes when the sun scorches. Fishermen, and men and women tending irrigated fields, have no choice but to work in potentially infected waters and are scarcely inclined to hike to distant latrines when the need arises. Nor is any amount of health education, by itself, likely to overcome the sheer inconvenience of scrupulous sanitation in poor rural areas. "In easygoing Egypt," writes Richard Critchfield, a journalist who has lived in rural Egypt, "it has proved easier to build the pyramids, feed the Roman Empire, and rule over medieval Islam than to keep the kids out of the water."

Obviously, no single control method can undo the threat of schistosomiasis. However, experience in several countries has proven that appropriate combinations of available measures can conquer this scourge. China's combined use of snail destruction, drug treatment, and rudimentary sanitation, and Puerto Rico's mixture of snail control and sanitation improvements have both brought dramatic results.

In Egypt, molluscicides used in tandem with drug therapy in the oasis region of Fayoum have pushed the prevalence of infection among the area's one million people down from 47 percent in 1969 to 8 percent in 1975—providing the country's first major success against its special curse. The isolation of this area, where all water comes from one canal, makes snail control there easier than it is in the labyrinthine canal networks of the Nile Delta, but Egyptian officials nonetheless hope to repeat the success in some other parts of the country.[12]

While available control measures leave much to be desired, a technology gap is not the real impediment to global progress against schistosomiasis. Where adequate resources are made available—a political, not a technical problem—the existing panoply of weapons is usually sufficient to make inroads against the disease. Unfortunately, control programs are usually expensive, costing from $0.40 to $12.00 per person per year in control areas.[13] In comparison, the national budget for *all* medical care is little more than a dollar per person in many poor countries. The need for cheap environmental control measures with one-time costs speaks for itself, as does the need for all-out efforts to prevent the further *spread* of schistosomiasis as water resources are developed.

The vast expansion of irrigated agriculture now being initiated throughout the Middle East, Southeast Asia, Africa, and Latin America poses a monumental public health challenge. The record of the past few decades of water resource development is not encouraging. Dr. B. B. Waddy, who has studied the health impact of reservoir development in several countries, notes that national governments, private developers, and international aid agencies have all repeated avoidable mistakes "with monotonous regularity."[14]

Signs of progress can be discerned. Following the extensive publicity accorded the larger-scale health debacles such as that caused by the Aswan High Dam, major aid agencies and most governments now usually consider the snail factor as they plan new water investments. The more blatant errors in the past, such as the siting of latrines right over irrigation canals in one African project, are unlikely to be repeated. But, on the other hand, irrigation developments by private investors or contractors are seldom scrutinized as carefully for possible environmental backlash as projects sponsored by major international agencies now are.

Health-conscious engineers have devised numerous measures for use in preventing the automatic spread of schistosomiasis into new tropical water-developments. New villages for people displaced by reservoirs can be located far from the water's edge or next to steep, snail-free banks. Irrigation canals can be lined, covered, or designed to produce a water flow too fast for the snails to survive in. Irrigation systems can employ pipes and avoid canals altogether. And, above all, the provision of potable water and sewage facilities can be regarded as an essential component of irrigation development. As Dr. Patricia Rosenfield observes, transforming people's landscapes without simultaneously transforming the sanitary conditions of their daily lives "is like placing a shoe on one foot and leaving the other one bare."[15]

Many effective means of fighting schistosomiasis are known. How seriously they will be considered by economic planners remains an open question. The benefits of new dams, more food, and more electric power are visible and measurable; they bring political credit to those in power, and they boost the GNP. Increases in the prevalence of schistosomiasis are, in contrast, nearly invisible and are confined to the politically powerless rural poor. For now, then, it appears inevitable that schistosomiasis will continue to spread, and at more than a snail's pace.

10. The Family Planning Factor

Pure water, a sanitary environment, and nutritious food have long been recognized as prerequisites of good health. In recent decades, medical studies have revealed another health essential—family planning. Women who bear children too early or too late in life, women who bear too many children, and women who bear children too close together endanger themselves and their children. Yet, even with knowledge of these hazards, most governments still do not provide all prospective parents—whether teenagers in Detroit or newlyweds in rural Ethiopia—with access to reliable contraception. Today, no health program can be considered complete unless it offers ready access to appropriate family-planning measures for all potential parents.[1]

No one can say for sure how many deaths and how much disease the universal availability and wise use of family-planning services could prevent. But it is known that some of the world's least fortunate women are twenty to thirty times more likely than their more privileged counterparts to die in childbirth. Infant mortality rates, always far higher than maternal mortality rates, also vary among societies by a factor of nearly twenty. Along with undernutrition and poor sanitation, the failure to prevent high-risk pregnancies contributes to the appallingly high mortality rates of mothers and children among the world's poor.

It is an unfortunate evolutionary fact that women become fertile several years before what is, for both mother and child, the safest time for birth; moreover, they usually remain fertile for ten to fifteen years beyond the period of lowest risk. While the onset of fertility ranges from age ten to the mid-teens, pregnancy becomes safest from a biological point of view around age twenty. The period of maximum safety lasts for about a decade; then, when a woman reaches the age of about thirty, risks to mother and child begin to rise and they continue to escalate with the mother's age.

The absolute size of these risks primarily reflects social and environmental conditions: a forty-two-year-old Swedish woman faces a lower hazard from giving birth than does a twenty-four-year-old woman in rural Pakistan, and deaths in pregnancy and childbirth among white women in the United States occur only one-third as frequently as those among nonwhite American women. But within every society and at every socioeconomic level, the odds that the mother or her child will succumb to death or disease increase when the mother gives birth too early or too late in her life.[2]

From 10 to 15 percent of all births in the world—some twelve to eighteen million a year—involve teenage mothers. For both biological and social reasons, many of these women are too young to be ideal mothers. Young mothers, their bodies often not wholly mature, face extra dangers in childbirth and are considerably more likely than mothers in their twenties to give birth to frail babies. The psychological perils of teenage pregnancy may be even greater than the biological hazards. Whether a teenage girl makes a fit parent depends upon her own emotional, financial, and educational resources, and upon the way her culture prepares and treats young mothers. But most fourteen- or fifteen-year-old girls lack the maturity and the means of support needed to give a baby a stable, healthful, and stimulating environment.[3]

Early pregnancy takes an even higher toll among babies

than among their adolescent mothers. A recent Pan American Health Organization (PAHO) survey of infant deaths in the Americas showed irrefutably that teenage pregnancy entails heightened risks for the newborn. In São Paulo, Brazil, for example, 104 of every thousand babies born to teenage mothers died before their first birthdays, compared with only fifty-three per thousand born to mothers between the ages of twenty-five and twenty-nine.[4]

In both poorer and richer countries, the increased tendency for the babies of teenagers to be born premature or underweight raises the infants' chances of early death. These babies succumb more readily than robust infants to infectious diseases and undernutrition. Among Californians, the PAHO survey revealed, twenty-six of every thousand infants born to mothers under age twenty died in their first year of life, compared to fifteen per thousand born to mothers in their late twenties. In Iran, where women marry young and bear children early, the high death rate among the babies of young mothers is reflected in a proverb: "The first two," it goes, "are for the crows."[5]

The proportion of all babies born to teenage mothers varies considerably among countries and does not correlate directly to income levels. In part, the proportion does reflect the customary age of marriage for girls. Although modernization seems to be gradually boosting average marriage ages the world over, especially among urban populations, girls in parts of many poor countries still normally marry while in their midteens. From 10 to 20 percent of the babies in most poor countries have teenage mothers.[6]

But marriage age alone does not determine the proportion of teenage to adult pregnancies. In the United States, for example, teenagers give birth to one-fifth of all infants—a ratio higher than that found in most poor countries. Since the average age of U.S. women when they first marry is 21 and rising, the explanation for this ratio involves more than the number of early marriages. Although birth rates among adult women have dropped steadily in recent years, the teenage birth rate has declined scarcely at all. In fact, among girls under fifteen years old, it has risen slightly. Thus, births to teenagers account for a higher and higher percentage of total births in the United States. A full third of the teenage births —200,000 every year—involve unwed mothers, and only the widespread availability of abortion services keeps the number that low. The rising number of births to unmarried teenagers presents a serious health problem, not to mention an enormous social challenge. The United States has plainly failed to reach teenagers with the information and wherewithal they need to avoid unwanted pregnancies. With sexual activity among teenagers on the increase, many family-planning officials fear that the number of teenage pregnancies can only increase.[7]

Women who become pregnant after their prime reproductive years have passed also take on added health risks for both themselves and their infants. Though maternal death rates are quite low in North America and Europe for all except women over forty, U.S. data from 1974 show that the incidence of deaths associated with pregnancy and childbirth among American women climbs steeply after mothers pass age thirty—rising from a low of ten maternal deaths per hundred thousand births among women in their early twenties to eighty-six per hundred thousand among women in their early forties, and then to 234 per hundred thousand among women over forty-five. (In comparison, in 1973 auto accidents claimed the lives of about twelve per hundred thousand U.S. women aged thirty to forty-four.)[8]

In poor countries, maternal risk also climbs dramatically with age. In Thailand, for instance, maternal death rates rise from 154 deaths per hundred thousand births among women in their twenties to 474 per hundred thousand among women in their forties. In parts of Bangladesh, more than 800 per hundred thousand women giving birth in their forties die as a result, compared to a grim enough maternal mortality rate of 380 per hundred thousand births among women in their early twenties.[9]

Once women pass the age of thirty, their odds of bearing a premature or underweight baby begin to rise along with their chances of experiencing complications during childbirth. Infant mortality rates also rise, though they remain lower than those for babies of teenage mothers.

Dangers other than maternal or infant death also surround late pregnancy. Older mothers are more likely than younger mothers to bear babies with congenital defects. The clearest rise in genetic risk involves the condition called Down's syndrome, commonly known as mongolism, whose victims suffer idiocy and physical disabilities. The incidence of mongolism among infants rises exponentially with the mother's age—ranging from near zero among the babies of young mothers to as many as fourteen mongoloids per thousand infants born to mothers over the age of forty, with the exact rate varying by country.[10] Today, many older women with access to sophisticated medical services take advantage of a new technique called amniocentesis that can identify certain congenital defects in the fetus. Many women choose abortion when Down's syndrome is discovered.

The number of children a woman bears in her life affects her health significantly. Her first birth carries a slightly higher risk of complications or death for her than the next two births do. Then, with the fourth birth, the incidences of maternal death, stillbirth, and infant and even childhood mortality begin to rise, jumping sharply with the birth of the fifth and every succeeding child.[11] Beyond a certain point, then, practice does not make perfect in childbearing; quite the contrary, it entails escalating dangers.

Since a woman's fifth and subsequent births involve extra

risks for mother and child regardless of the woman's social level, some basic biological laws appear to be involved. Socio-economic factors, however, are the overwhelming determinants of risks posed by high fertility. By far the strongest negative health impact of large families appears among the world's lowest income groups—and many impoverished women in Africa, Asia, and Latin America bear more than five children each. In Rwanda, 20 percent of all infants who are the fifth-born in their families die within a year of birth. Among the ninth-born and succeeding children, the risk of death is doubled: 40 percent die by age one.[12]

Studies throughout the world have consistently shown that children in large, poor families run a heightened risk of suffering from undernutrition (and hence of succumbing to disease and death). These nutritional studies go a long way toward explaining why the number of children born to a woman affects the survival odds of her young children as well as of her infants. Not surprisingly, the diets of all the members of large, poor families tend to be poorer than those of members of smaller families with comparable incomes. The latest-born children are usually hardest hit, sometimes in part because of discrimination (especially against females) in family food distribution, but also because they must live on reduced average portions during their nutritionally vulnerable early years. In Congo, for example, members of families with four or fewer members consume an average of about three thousand calories each per day; those in families larger than nine eat an average of only two thousand calories per day. Doctors in Hyderabad, India, recently found that 61 percent of all the severely undernourished children they saw were of the fourth or later birth order. The doctors calculate that even without any other improvements in income, food availability, or medical care, the "limitation of family size to three children would bring down the incidence of the severe forms of protein-calorie malnutrition by at least 60 percent."[13]

The ill effects of numerous births on both mothers and their children are most pronounced when the intervals between these births are short. A study in Punjab, India, showed that infants born less than two years after the previous child were 50 percent more likely to die by age one than were infants born two to four years after the previous child. During the 1960s in Guayaquil, Ecuador, fifty-eight per thousand babies born within one to two years of their predecessors died by their first birthdays; the comparable death rate among babies born three to four years after a sibling was thirty-seven per thousand.[14]

A short interval between births holds dangers for the next youngest child too. When another baby appears quickly, the nursing child may be preemptively weaned, and there may not be enough food to replace fully the mother's milk. The word "kwashiorkor" (the name of the childhood protein-deficiency disease) literally means "the disease of the deposed baby when the next one is born." In the Ga language of Ghana from which it is drawn, the word carries a connotation of sibling rivalry as well as of sickness.[15]

A rapid succession of pregnancies can weaken or even kill a woman, as well her offspring. A poorly fed woman is in greatest danger, for pregnancy and lactation both exact nutritional costs that poor women are seldom able to offset by eating more and better food. When pregnant, a moderately active, well-fed woman needs roughly three hundred calories per day more than she otherwise would. When nursing, she needs an even larger dietary supplement to maintain her health.[16]

For millions of African, Asian, and Latin American women, teenage marriage is followed by two decades or more of nearly uninterrupted pregnancy and lactation from which they never have a chance to recuperate. During these taxing decades, moreover, women are often saddled with much of the agricultural work and with other strenuous tasks such as firewood gathering and water carrying—duties that mothers frequently carry out with their youngest infants strapped on their backs.

Throughout the poor countries one sees women in their thirties with the haggard, wizened faces and bodies of the aged, victims of what Dr. Derrick B. Jelliffe has called the "maternal depletion syndrome." Undernourished, often anemic, and generally enervated by the biological burdens of excessive reproduction, the victims of this syndrome become increasingly vulnerable to death during childbirth or to simple infectious diseases at any time. Their babies swell the infant mortality statistics.[17]

When contraceptives are not available, are not used, or fail (as all available methods sometimes do), a growing share of the world's women are unwilling to go through with an unplanned pregnancy. Some 35–55 million pregnancies are terminated each year by induced abortion. When performed early in a pregnancy by trained personnel, abortion involves considerably less risk for a woman than pregnancy and childbirth do. In the developed countries, legal abortions in the first three months of pregnancy are less than one-fourth as likely to cause maternal death than are pregnancy and childbirth.[18] Legal abortion's comparative health advantage over childbearing in poor countries has not been documented; but given the far higher risks involved in childbearing in such places, it is probably even larger.

About two-thirds of all women now live in countries where abortion is either legal or carries no threat of criminal prosecution.[19] Although low-income women often lack the means or knowledge to take advantage of legal and safe abortions and though medical establishments in many lands cannot meet the demand for legal abortions, many women in relatively affluent or progressive countries can easily obtain expert operations. Even where abortion is illegal, wealthy women can usually find doctors willing to perform safe abortions clandestinely or can travel abroad to get legal operations. But for millions of women who live in countries where abortion is legally proscribed or who lack access to expert abortions, conditions are less favorable. Some must trust the hands of unskilled practitioners, and some, in desperation, try to perform abortions upon themselves using crude means.

An inexpert abortion involves a high risk of complications and death for a woman. Since such abortions are usually performed illegally and secretly, no one has measured precisely the risks they involve. But the health consequences of poorly done abortions cannot escape notice. Hospitals in many countries where abortion is illegal are besieged with the victims of inexpert abortionists, and efforts to salvage the lives of these unlucky women absorb precious medical resources. According to the Bolivian Ministry of Public Health, the treatment of complications from illegal abortions accounts for more than 60 percent of Bolivia's obstetrical and gynecological expenditures. Twenty-four percent of the deaths in the El Salvador Maternity Hospital result from illegal abortions; during the 1960s, half of the maternity-related deaths in Santiago, Chile, followed illegal abortions. A 1964 study in Cali, Colombia, found that abortion complications were the leading cause of death among females between the ages of fifteen and thirty-five. In California in the 1960s, before the abortion law was liberalized, complications arising from illegal abortions accounted for one in five of the state's maternal deaths, most of which struck low-income women.[20]

Where abortion is illegal, women pay with their lives. In 1966, after a decade with a liberal abortion law, Romania took the unusual step of reversing its policies and severely limiting the availability of abortions. As the government had hoped, the birth rate jumped—but so too did the number of maternal deaths associated with illegal abortions. Although the total number of abortions performed in Romania undoubtedly fell between 1964 and 1972, the number of reported maternal deaths arising from post-abortion complications more than quadrupled, rising from eighty-three to 370.[21]

Few people consider abortion an ideal means of fertility control. Improving sex education and making contraceptives available to all, regardless of ability to pay, are alternative means of reducing the number of unwanted births. Even where such services are provided, however, unwanted pregnancies still occur. Neither the available means of contraception nor human forethought is perfectly reliable. Abortions will take place regardless of how the laws read; an unavoidable issue, then, is whether the lives of women are to be jeopardized by unrealistic laws.

The health risks associated with the lack of family planning are well established, but what health risks does contraception involve? Of all contraceptive methods, the birth-control pill has generated the hottest controversy. The side effects and the occasional deaths linked to pill use have received extensive media coverage. However, the hazards of the pill, like those of any threat, can be meaningfully measured only against the hazards of alternatives—in this case, the risks involved either in uncontrolled fertility or in the use of other means of contraception.

Such comparisons dramatize a crucial fact: all common methods of contraception, including the pill, entail fewer health risks than do pregnancy and childbirth. The only known exception concerns women over forty in developed countries; for them, using oral contraceptives may involve a mortality risk slightly higher than the risk associated with childbearing—especially if they are cigarette smokers. But for women under forty, and for women of all ages using any means of contraception but the pill, practicing contraception is safer than becoming pregnant and giving birth.[22] (These data should not, of course, engender complacency about the health problems related to contraception. Moreover, until an entire generation of pill-using women live out their lives, the record on the long-term effects of the pill will be incomplete.)

Although the relative safety of practicing contraception compared to childbearing has been established only for developed Western countries, the difference is undoubtedly even greater in poor countries, where the dangers associated with childbirth are so high. Using particular contraceptives such as the intrauterine device (IUD), which has been associated with increased blood loss in menstruation and also with infection, may be more dangerous for women living in an environment of poverty than for affluent women who have access to good medical care. Some researchers also believe that birth-control pills might accentuate certain nutrient deficiencies in undernourished women (the significance of this potential effect is now being investigated by the World Health Organization and by the U.S. Agency for International Development, but results are not yet available). At the same time, considerable evidence indicates that pill use may ameliorate other nutritional problems such as iron-deficiency anemia. Furthermore, some doctors suggest that the pill may actually be safer for women in poor than in rich countries: because of dietary or other lifestyle differences, women in poor countries tend to be less susceptible to the cardiovascular problems that pill use sometimes exacerbates.[23]

Disparities in the comparative safety of different contraceptives do, of course, exist. A realistic assessment of contraceptive risks should take into account the deaths associated with pregnancy and childbirth when contraceptives fail, as well as any deaths caused directly by the method. In addition, the risks associated with abortion, whether used as the primary birth-control method or as a back-up measure in cases of contraceptive failure, should also be weighed.

Such a comprehensive assessment of relative risks reveals that, though the pill is apparently quite safe for younger women, the IUD is even safer for women of all ages in developed countries. Neither the diaphragm nor the condom involves any health hazard in itself at all, but these devices are less reliable and more difficult to use than the pill or the IUD. However, condom or diaphragm use, when combined with legal, early abortion as a back-up measure, offers the safest means (short of sterilization) of achieving 100-percent-effective fertility control.[24]

When safe abortion is not available and childbearing risks are high, the methods that carry the lowest overall risks are those that provide the surest contraception—that is, the pill and the IUD. For example, an estimated 23,000 women died as a consequence of pregnancy and childbirth in Pakistan in 1975, about ten thousand of whom probably died from complications associated with induced abortions. "Had all 23,000 been users of the pill," calculates Dr. Andrew P. Haynal, "only one would have died due to the method and another in pregnancy resulting from method failure."[25]

The marginal mortality risk associated with the use of one or another contraceptive is important; but seldom is it the sole consideration guiding most couples' or women's decisions about birth control. The need for the psychological security born of the pill's near-total effectiveness, appreciation of the convenience of pills or IUDs compared to diaphragms or condoms, or the unwillingness to abort unplanned pregnancies leads some women to pick the pill or the IUD. Conversely, some women reject the pill because of physical side effects that are not reflected in the mortality statistics. Others find the uncertainty about the long-term health effects of the pill to be a persuasive reason for avoiding its use.

Only as they approach forty should most women turn to methods of birth control other than the pill strictly on the basis of available medical evidence. Correlations of pill use in developed countries to an increased risk of cardiovascular disorders such as heart attacks and blood clots suggest that women of any age who are especially susceptible to these diseases—those who smoke or who have high blood cholesterol, high blood pressure, or diabetes—should also strongly consider alternatives to the pill. Cigarette smoking and pill use appear to combine to boost heart-disease risks dramatically; and, in fact, women who smoke account for a highly disproportionate share of pill-associated cardiovascular deaths. For smokers, pill use even before age forty may be more hazardous than childbearing; for nonsmokers, pill use after age forty may be safer than childbearing. Because the pill may be linked to the genesis of rare, nonmalignant liver tumors, doctors now recommend that women with liver problems should also not take the pill.[26]

Sterilization is growing in popularity around the world among individuals who wish to remain childless or to have no more children. Quite safe for both women and men, sterilization operations afford adults complete peace of mind on the subject of contraception. Of every hundred thousand forty-year-old women in developed countries who undergo tubal sterilizations, from fifteen to thirty, or less than .03 percent, die as a consequence of the operation, and newly developed operating procedures are steadily reducing the risks. In contrast, roughly 120 of every hundred thousand women who begin using the pill at age forty and continue to use it to the end of their fertile years can be expected to die as a result of pill use; and women using no contraception at age forty and beyond face a similarly high risk of maternity-related death. Vasectomies are even safer than tubal sterilizations—in fact, they are the safest means of birth control known, with the possible exception of abstinence. Although postoperative infections have reportedly caused some deaths in India, no vasectomy-associated deaths have ever been reported in developed countries.[27]

The ideal contraceptive would be undetectable, reversible, simple and convenient to use, certain in effect, and absolutely safe. No existing contraceptive meets this bill, a fact that accentuates the urgency of research on new contraceptives for both men and women. Nevertheless, available contraceptives do offer choices that can promote better health.

Clearly, general health would improve markedly if family-planning measures were more widely available and more widely used to reduce early and late pregnancies, to limit family sizes, and to keep a healthy interval between births. Examining data from around the world, Dorothy Nortman of the Population Council has calculated the health benefits for women that would result if births in the risky early and late periods of female fertility were eliminated. "If women had births only in the age interval 20–34," she writes, "maternal mortality would come down by 19 percent in Mexico, Thailand, Venezuela, and the United States; by 23 percent in Colombia and France; and by 25 percent in the Philippines."[28]

Nicholas H. Wright estimates that if each woman in the United States were to bear no more than three children, and were to bear them only when she is between the ages of twenty and thirty-four, deaths among infants would be reduced by 29 percent nationally. In Thailand, the 27 percent reduction in infant mortality that would follow a limitation of births to four per woman, all to mothers between the ages of twenty and thirty-four, would mean that about 60,000 fewer infant deaths would occur each year.[29]

The interaction of poverty and excessive fertility produces a self-reinforcing cycle of desperation: expecting that some of their offspring will not survive to adulthood, parents may feel compelled to produce more babies than they want. In Rwanda, the average thirty-year-old woman has given birth seven times in her twelve years of marriage, but only five of her children will survive to adulthood. Similarly, because of high rates of fetal loss and infant mortality, women in India must become pregnant eight times to raise five children.[30] Numerous births, numerous infant and child deaths, and strain on the health of surviving family members all flow almost inexorably from unlimited fertility combined with poverty.

But, if economic and social policies aimed at pushing down mortality rates and at creating a general climate of social progress can be enacted, the negative cycle of poverty and fertility can perhaps be halted. In its place, a positive cycle could take hold. Parents, more confident that their children will survive to adulthood, may become more receptive to family-planning advice. Families in turn could enjoy the further health benefits accruing from a health-promoting childbearing pattern.

Giving every person the knowledge and means to manage her or his fertility would have social benefits beyond the direct improvement of health. These include, for example, the psychological security that reliable contraception affords couples and the economic security that having no unwanted children affords families. For women especially, a major benefit is the ability to pursue educational or career plans without the disruption of an unplanned pregnancy. Furthermore, to the extent that individuals follow the safest reproductive pattern, the national birth rate—and hence the population growth rate—would drop considerably in many countries.

Educating people about the health benefits of family planning is one task that governments can undertake to encourage an optimal reproductive pattern for all families. Indeed, young people's preparation for life is not complete unless they are thoroughly versed in the facts of health, sexuality, and fertility control. Other more specific policies can also further that goal. Raising the age of marriage through legislation and exhortation, as the Chinese have done, can curb the incidence of early pregnancies. Where births out of wedlock are common (as they are in the Americas), however, changing the legal age of marriage will not by itself solve the problem of teenage pregnancy.

Governments can assure that various contraceptives are universally available at a cost all can afford. They can drastically cut the health costs of abortion by making it legal and by ensuring that all women, regardless of their ability to pay, have access to safe abortions. The increasing tendency for those who have attained their desired family size to turn to sterilization as a safe and permanent means of contraception also deserves encouragement on health grounds.

At the same time, research on contraceptive alternatives and safety deserves far greater support. A recent study commissioned by the Ford Foundation concluded that the current global research expenditure on fertility control and contraceptive safety comprises less than 2 percent of governmental medical research allocations in the nineteen countries for which data are available. In order "to exploit adequately existing knowledge and opportunities" in this field, global research funds devoted to contraception need to be tripled to at least $361 million (in 1976 dollars)—still less than half of what the United States alone spends on cancer research. Because of the uncertain profit-making potential of contraceptive research, the report observes, private corporations are not filling this social gap. Only governments can make the needed commitment.[31]

At the first World Population Conference, a gathering of scientists organized by family-planning pioneer Margaret Sanger and held in Geneva in 1927, the controversial topic of contraception was barred from the agenda by uneasy delegates.[32] Decades of medical research and social change have, however, wrought a massive shift in attitudes. At the U.N. World Population Conference in Bucharest in 1974, the nations of the world collectively agreed that "all couples and individuals have the basic right to decide freely and responsibly the number and spacing of their children and to have the information, education and means to do so." Implementing this goal would immediately improve personal health, even as it laid the groundwork for meeting other long-term social challenges associated with rapid population growth. Making family-planning services (including legal abortion) universally available will certainly not in itself solve the acute health problems of the world's poor; until this condition is met, however, no other combination of policies is likely to solve them either. Like pure water, like nutritious food, family planning is essential to good health.

11. *Creating Better Health*

No SOCIETY has deactivated both traditional and modern environmental health threats. Today's more developed societies have markedly cut the toll of traditional disease killers, but they have also created lifestyles and technologies that entail new health risks. Meanwhile, more than a third of humanity must contend daily with age-old scourges. Some unfortunates must cope with both ancient and modern threats.

How would a society that made human health a top priority look? To begin with, in such a society the circumstances of conception and gestation would maximize the chances of each child being born robust and well equipped to survive the perilous early months, and of subsequently leading a long, healthy life. Through judicious family planning, women would avoid giving birth before or after their safest childbearing years, and none would bear large numbers of children. Since prospective mothers would consume well-balanced diets throughout their own lives and adequate dietary supplements during pregnancy, the number of premature or underweight births would be minimized. Pregnant women would not smoke, would not take potentially hazardous drugs, and would not be exposed to toxic chemicals or radiation on the job or at home.

Good sanitation would be a watchword; children's contacts with infectious agents and parasites would be limited, since everyone would live in clean residences with adequate pure water and sanitary sewage facilities close at hand. Nutritional basics would be universally understood; children would be raised on diets that encouraged neither undernutrition nor overnutrition and, from an early age, physical activity would be integral to daily life. Adults would eschew excess calories and fats in their diets, avoid heavy drinking, and get plenty of regular exercise. The number of potentially hazardous environmental agents in circulation would be slashed; only those chemicals that had been rigorously tested for long-term health effects would be added to foods and other products. Smoking would be considered antisocial, and the cigarette smoker would gradually become an extinct species. Workers' health would be strongly protected; if in some cases safeguards and vigilance in the workplace could not guarantee workers reasonable peace of mind about their health, consumers would simply do without particularly dangerous materials and products. Factories would spend what is necessary to eliminate hazardous pollutants. Only low-polluting vehicles would be allowed on roads; and, in urban centers, the widespread use of bicycles and public transportation would offset driving restrictions.

The life-giving properties of such a regime can be inferred, if not predicted precisely. Deaths among infants would be rare, disease deaths among children and young adults rarer still. Infectious diseases would certainly continue to afflict, occasionally fatally, people of all ages but in general would be neither frequent nor life-threatening. Polio, measles, diphtheria, and other diseases would be emasculated by the strategic use of vaccines.

Heart attacks and other cardiovascular conditions would probably take lives among the aged, but they would lose power over the many middle-aged men whose lives they threaten today. Some cancer cases would occur, but the general incidence of cancer would undoubtedly plummet from the levels now prevailing in developed countries. The health of many in middle and old age would improve even as the average length of life was extended. Far fewer people would be debilitated in their forties, fifties, and sixties by circulatory and other ailments than are today.

Beyond the amounts spent to prevent disease, medical expenditures would be concentrated on nonpreventable threats and on the special health (and social) problems of old age. Less money would be wasted trying to save people from ailments that could have been avoided in the first place. Whatever the amount it spent on health care, such a society would get more life for its money than is the rule anywhere today.

What obstacles now keep individuals from enjoying the best possible health? Certainly they are not technological. Achieving the ideal health conditions just described requires no new breakthroughs in medical research—though any that do occur might improve health still more. Nor do insurmountable genetic obstacles bar the way. To be sure, some diseases are inherited and thus not preventable. But only rarely is an individual's health defined by heredity; as the noted geneticist Theodosius Dobzhansky observed, "Genes determine not 'characters' or 'traits' but reactions or responses." Heredity influences individual susceptibilities to the diseases that take most lives today, but environmental factors usually determine whether that potential is realized.[1]

The true obstacles to better health, then, are political failures—failures of nations to organize affairs to minimize environmental health threats, and failures of individuals to avoid self-destructive lifestyles. Significant improvements in health require massive attacks on todays' major sources of disease: unjust social systems, skewed investment priorities, carelessly used technologies, and reckless personal behavior patterns.

In rich and poor societies, changes in both government policies and personal habits are essential to better health. Depending on their current health conditions, however, different societies must establish different priorities. In poorer countries, the biggest health gains will follow social reforms that reduce undernutrition and construction programs that provide people with clean water and sewage facilities. In more affluent countries, major health gains will necessarily involve habit-breaking. If cigarette smoking, overnutrition, and sedentary living remain widespread, neither the strictest controls of pollution and toxic chemicals nor the most elaborate medical facilities can improve the health picture much. If, through wise planning, developing countries can possibly avoid duplicating all the hazards now associated with industrialism and affluence even as they strive to eliminate traditional health hazards, they will give their people opportunities that money alone cannot buy.

A comparison of mortality rates around the world reveals what should be humankind's top health-care priority: cutting the number of infants and children lost to undernutrition and infectious disease. An estimated thirteen million children aged five and under die each year—about thirty-five thousand a day, so many that the power of the living to comprehend the deep daily tragedy has grown dull.

The medical communities in developing countries, where nearly all preventable childhood deaths occur, often fail to meet the simple health-care needs of the poor, especially the rural poor. Medical systems in many developing countries, critics observe, have tended to follow the organizational example of the West—with the result that modern hospitals and developed urban areas receive unjustifiable shares of scanty health resources.

While it underscores the need for a more equitable dissemination of medical resources, analysis of the disease prob-

lems of the poor tells us something more profound: that solving these problems has little to do with medical care per se.
Consider the experience of a hospital in Cali, Colombia, in
the 1960s. Its excellent modern unit for the care of premature
infants achieved in-hospital survival rates comparable to
those in North America. Yet 70 percent of the prematurely
born infants died within three months of their discharge
from the hospital nursery.[2]

Diseases rooted in the ecology of poverty can only be
conquered by eradicating their social and physical origins.
Major improvements in the health of the world's poorest half
will not be achieved with hospitals, doctors, and drugs, but
with wells, latrines, land reforms, small-farm credit programs, family planning, and community education. Health
strategies, of which medical care should constitute one component, must take account of the broad cultural and economic factors that influence nutritional and sanitary conditions.

The two absolute prerequisites of decent health are an
adequate supply of food and convenient access to abundant
quantities of reasonably pure water. When these two basic
needs are met, infant and childhood mortality inevitably
plummets. The potential outlines of national strategies to
fight undernutrition were sketched in Chapter 3, but it must
be reemphasized that undernutrition reflects far more than
a food-supply problem and prevails most often where incomes are extremely low or disparate. Even feeding programs aimed at disadvantaged groups cannot more than dent
a large-scale undernutrition problem. Development that increases the food production, employment prospects, and incomes of the rural and urban poor will scale down undernutrition; development that promotes economic inequality
may worsen it.

According to some estimates, the worldwide burden of
infectious diseases would shrink by as much as 80 percent if

everyone had access to safe water and made good use of it for proper sanitation.[3] Although providing those who lack them with adequate sanitary facilities is the cheapest and fastest way to improve human health, about one-third of humanity has yet to reap the benefits of the sanitary revolution that swept through Europe and North America in the late nineteenth century. Mobilized communities can improve local sanitation measurably, but the construction of safe water-supply and sewage-disposal (or recycling) systems also requires money and some expertise. And, as a comparison of the funds devoted to sanitary improvements with those lavished on other purposes demonstrates, those who control the world's purses have been only half-heartedly committed to better health.

In 1976, the World Health Organization set what it believes are realistic global sanitation targets for 1980. WHO hopes to prod nations into spending $35 billion over five years to boost the percentage of the developing-country population with ready access to safe water from 29 to 38 percent, and the portion with safe sewage disposal from 25 to 32 percent.[4] Even if these targets are met, however, the total spent to achieve them will constitute less than one-fortieth of global military expenditures during the same period; or, to make what may be a more apt comparison, the funds spent to save lives by constructing water and sewage facilities will constitute less than one-twelfth of the money consumers will have spent on cigarettes during those years. Yet, since the targets are modest and since population growth will cancel out some gains, the absolute number of people lacking basic sanitary services will scarcely be reduced by 1980 in any case.

Family planning services are a third important contributor to good health. At the individual level, uncontrolled fertility directly threatens the well-being of mothers and infants. At the community level, it can undermine even the strongest efforts to wipe out environmental disease-promoters. When populations double every twenty-five or thirty years, as they now do in some countries, constructing safe water and sewage facilities becomes a Sisyphean task. Stepping up food production fast enough also presents a stiff order; and, in some areas, mounting population pressures, manifested in deforestation, the extension of farming onto marginal lands, and overgrazing, actually impair the land's capacity to support life. Temporary rises in death rates in several areas of Asia and Africa in the early 1970s, apparently a consequence of heightened nutritional stress, may well have portended greater tragedies to come.[5]

Family planning will not solve basic development and equity problems, but it is an essential component of social progress. Widely and wisely used, contraception can better the welfare of the present generation as it betters the prospects of future generations, who will have to cope with the environment we bequeath them. Family planning is most apt to be practiced in a climate of economic progress, especially when the survival odds of infants and children are fast improving. But a large share of the more than 300 million couples who do not use contraception lack even the choice, for they cannot obtain reliable contraceptives.[6]

The Chinese system of "barefoot doctors"—men and women with minimal formal medical training who provide rudimentary health services and encourage cleanliness and family planning in their own communities—has recently received much acclaim. These health promoters usually do in fact wear shoes or sandals, but their involvement with their fellow citizens is, as their nickname suggests, unostentatious. Aspects of the Chinese medical-care experience deserve to be emulated in rich as well as in poor countries. At the same time, of course, the underlying sources of China's health progress should be held in mind. Effective "medical" auxiliaries work two jobs. Besides providing vaccines, antibiotics, and safe abortions, they do environmental work and teach their clients how to prevent disease. And, perhaps most important, such health agents have the greatest impact where the broader social prerequisites of good health are met.

In addition to barefoot doctors, poor countries need "barefoot water engineers" who can cheaply provide moderately pure water supplies instead of the more sophisticated and expensive water systems that professional engineers prefer to build.[7] They also need "barefoot agricultural-extension agents" who will advise the struggling small-scale farmers as well as the big landowners who customarily receive most available services and credit. Perhaps the greatest need of all is for "barefoot economists" and "barefoot politicians" who will work for economic reforms that give the dispossessed a chance to better their lot and who will value life above abstract growth indicators.

In rich countries, as in poor ones, further significant gains in health will depend less upon medical science than upon broader social changes. The spiraling cost of medical care in the West is a complex social issue in its own right; but today's massive disease-control expenditures bear surprisingly little relation to overall health trends, except insofar as part of these funds could be better spent on disease prevention. While costly procedures such as organ transplants, the use of artificial kidneys, and heroic efforts to save cancer victims boost medical bills and save some individual lives, they affect the basic health picture only marginally. Funds poured into curative systems in developed countries have reached the point of rapidly diminishing returns.

The limits to the benefits of a costly disease-treatment system are suggested by the American experience. During 1975, American health expenditures *grew* by more than a billion dollars a month, adding up to an annual total of $115 billion. One twelfth of the U.S. national product is now devoured by the medical-care system. Yet American life ex-

pectancy is years below and infant mortality is well above the
rates prevailing in several European countries where per
capita medical expenditures average much less. Although
billions of dollars have been spent over the decades on medical research and curative techniques, a white American male
of seventy can expect to live only *one year* longer—to age
eighty—than could his counterpart at the beginning of the
century.[8]

To be sure, health conditions in today's more developed
countries shine by any historical standard. Although potential lifespans for those surviving childhood have not been
extended much, more people are living long lives than ever
before. Yet, each year millions of people in developed countries die or grow infirm unnecessarily early. In the early
1970s, nearly four of every ten deaths in the United States
and Japan involved victims under the age of sixty-five; and
nearly three in ten deaths in France and the Federal Repub-
lic of Germany occurred among those under sixty-five.

The historical statistics of health progress offer little comfort to the parents of a child smitten by leukemia, the woman
widowed at age forty by her husband's heart attack, or the
youngster whose mother is carried off by cancer. In developed countries today, preventing deaths and debilities
among the young and among the middle-aged should over-
ride all other health goals. The same measures that bring
down the death and disease toll among middle-aged people
will also prolong old age and salve its physical sting, since the
seeds of many of the chronic diseases that torment and kill
the aged are sown early in life.

To the extent that an ounce of prevention is worth a
pound of cure, children and young adults should receive
much more attention than their low death rates would suggest. An individual's health in middle and old age is largely
determined by personal habits formed and environmental
influences first felt in youth. The heart attacks that fell the

unsuspecting are usually the culmination of decades of dietary excesses, physical inactivity, and cigarette smoking. So too the smoking and eating habits and the occupational and other exposures to carcinogens that engender fatal cancers are cumulative in their effects.

Personal lifestyles constitute one of the strategic frontiers of preventive medicine in developed countries today. "It can be said unequivocally that a significant reduction in sedentary living and overnutrition, alcoholism, hypertension, and excessive cigarette smoking would save more lives in the age range forty to sixty-four than the best current medical practice," three prominent U.S. medical researchers recently wrote.[9]

By studying the lives of seven thousand men and women in California, Drs. Nedra B. Belloc and Lester Breslow have assembled eye-opening evidence of the health importance of personal habits. They correlated both physical well-being and lifespans to adherence to seven basic practices:

1) sleeping seven to eight hours each night;
2) eating three meals a day at regular times with little snacking;
3) eating breakfast every day;
4) maintaining desirable body weight;
5) avoiding excessive alcohol consumption;
6) getting regular exercise;
7) not smoking

Belloc and Breslow write that "the physical health status of those reported following all seven good health practices was consistently about the same as those thirty years younger who followed few or none of these practices." They found, moreover, that whereas men at age forty-five who follow three or fewer of these practices can expect to live to sixty-seven, those following six or seven of the practices can expect to live to seventy-eight. Similarly, they found that forty-five-year-old women who follow six or seven of the health prac-

tices push their average age of death to eighty-one, while
women who abide by three or fewer of the practices can
expect to die at seventy-four.[10]

Relating behavior, health, and public policy poses profound philosophical questions. Almost everyone would grant
an individual the prerogative of choosing a lifestyle that implicitly subordinates personal health to other values. Most
would also assign to the individual some responsibility for
personal actions. At the same time, psychologists have
proven how strongly the social environment can influence
personal behavior; and the line between personal prerogative and personal responsibility to fellow citizens is not easily
drawn.

How relevant is the notion of individual responsibility
when teenagers become addicted to nicotine after seeing
their parents, teachers, and possibly even their doctors smoking? How can the children of the Age of Advertising be
expected to blind themselves to images of cigarettes as
agents of liberation and sexual attractiveness? Can overnutrition be attributed solely to lack of willpower when infants are
overfed from birth, when schools teach nothing about the
suspected dangers of high-fat diets, and when national leaders speak in favor of subsidies to those who produce butter
and eggs?

Not only do most societies fail to educate themselves
about the prerequisites of better health; all too often government agricultural policies, tax policies, and other programs
support unhealthy lifestyles. It is no affront to individual dig-
nity to suggest that social and economic policies that encourage self-destructive habits should be altered or that advertising on behalf of potentially dangerous products be curbed.
Nor need governments hesitate to underwrite programs and
economic incentives that promote life-saving personal habits. The molding of a social milieu that promotes enlightened
self-interest is not a public infringement on personal rights,
but rather a public responsibility to the individual.

If societies have a collective responsibility to build a health-promoting climate, do individuals have, in turn, a social responsibility to try to protect their own health? One's answer to this question depends largely on one's basic assumptions about the purposes of social organization. To the extent that personal behavior infringes on the well-being of others, however, the question of personal responsibility to the community may be reduced in part to a comparatively simple question of fairness. And, as Dr. John H. Knowles has written, "one man's freedom in health is another man's shackle in taxes and insurance premiums."[11] As health-care burdens around the world are increasingly borne by collective groups, whether by those who join health insurance programs or by those who pay for public doctors and hospitals, the finances of medical equity deserve new attention. One way or another, people who act to protect their own health subsidize those who don't. Those who live dangerously—not to mention those who encourage and profit from people's unhealthy habits—account for disproportionate shares of society's health costs, and they must be made to foot a just share of the medical bills.

Eliminating some health threats, of course, lies far beyond the power of the individual acting alone. Only collective behavioral changes and effective public policies can hold down air and water pollution or free workplaces and homes of dangerous substances. A lone individual forsaking his automobile cannot eradicate photochemical smog; radical changes in car design and alterations in a whole city's commuting habits perhaps can. Similarly, a factory worker who handles carcinogenic materials lacks both the scientific knowledge to identify his danger and the political power needed to force corporations to invest in protective technologies.

As both logic and economics suggest, the best way to deal with the health threats posed by modern industrial processes is to prevent them. Pollution can be reduced, deadly substances can be identified and avoided, and the uses of harmful chemicals can be carefully restricted. So long as these tacks fail or remain untried, however, ways must be devised to distribute more equitably the costs of dangerous production patterns. At a minimum, all who initiate or profit by hazardous activities must be forced to compensate generously those who suffer as a result of such activities.

Production that imperils workers or the community is often allowed to continue because its social "benefit" is judged to outweigh the ensuing risks. Seldom, however, do those who enjoy the major benefits face the greatest risks. To date, moreover, no satisfactory means has been devised for ascribing values to either the benefits or the risks involved in a particular production process. How do we determine the social value, as opposed to the market value, of a product, particularly of one that neither survival nor comfort requires? And, apart from the obvious difficulty of appraising suffering and unnecessary death, how are the costs of health risks to be figured when, as is often the case, the magnitude of a given health hazard cannot be determined precisely? Shorn of economic and scientific terminology, benefit-risk calculations are political judgments that reflect assumptions about what things matter and how much these things are worth.

Though environmental-health priorities differ from one country to the next, the study of health conditions and trends everywhere turns up one basic truth: national economic growth and better health are not synonymous. "Too often is development equated with economic growth instead of with the progressive well-being of the people," says Dr. Halfdan Mahler, the Director-General of the World Health Organization.[12] Past transitions from low-income agrarian societies to high-income industrial ones have involved eventual transitions from poor to good sanitation and from shaky to abundant food supplies. Often, however, the wheels of change have unnecessarily crushed enormous numbers of humans. Dickens, Engels, and many others testified to the squalid living conditions during the initial decades of the Industrial Revolution, and the lot of the poor is voiced by equally astute social critics today.

In any case, today's poor countries are not simply recapitulating development as Europe and North America experienced it in the nineteenth or early twentieth centuries. Poor countries' economic and demographic plights are historically unique: far from conquering new territory, many of the countries were themselves colonized; and far from eager to welcome immigrants into their labor forces, they must cope with a population growth rate much higher than that ever reached in Europe or North America. Clearly, moreover, development as it is now unfolding in many low-income countries will not lead to the widely shared middle-class affluence of today's developed countries. Recent trends reveal that some kinds of "development" intensify economic inequality, stranding huge numbers in abysmally deep poverty. Unaccompanied by social reforms, economic growth may not only bypass some; it may grind them under its heel.

Brazil's recent development history provides a documented but by no means isolated example. The negative nutritional impact of Brazil's soybean-export boom, which has sent up the price of the food beans that provide the country's poor with their protein staple, fits into a broader pattern of widening income disparities. Between 1960 and 1970, the wealthiest 3.5 percent of Brazil's income-earning population increased their share of national income from one-fourth to one-third; simultaneously, the income share of the bottom 43 percent of earners fell from 11 percent to 8 percent of the total.[13]

The possible health consequences of such a development pattern are indicated by infant mortality data from São

Paulo, Brazil's slum-ringed modern industrial center. Bely-
ing both the global trend and the city's own experience in
the previous decade, São Paulo's infant mortality rate rose
from sixty deaths per thousand live births in 1961 to eighty-
nine deaths per thousand in 1970. The migration of impoverished peasants into the city undoubtedly boosted urban mortality figures; but, Dr. Walter Leser of São Paulo University
argues, migration rates were about the same in the 1950s and
the sixties, so migration alone probably does not explain the
health reversal. One abetting factor may well have been the
decline in the purchasing power of workers' minimum sala-
ries, which fell in real terms by 30 percent during the sixties.[14]

Whatever a country's income level, technological and economic changes that undermine health without providing
commensurate social benefits can occur. If "development" is
to mean an improvement in well-being, as most would agree
it should, then laissez-faire development isn't always development at all. Adam Smith's "invisible hand" appears as
loath to halt the unfortunate decline in breast feeding among
the poor as to ensure that new industrial chemicals are
thoroughly tested for carcinogenicity. Only a determined
polity can give priority to direct indicators of social well-
being, such as health and nutritional status, over misleading
indicators of progress such as baby bottle sales in Bolivia, or
the availability in the United States of unneeded plastic gim-
mickry whose production perils workers.[15]

All life forms are shaped by natural evolution and depend
upon the earth's basic biological, geological, and chemical
cycles for sustenance. *Homo sapiens,* however, is the first
species able and willing to alter nature's life-support systems
significantly, the first to become a dominant evolutionary
force in its own right.[16] Through extraction, production, and
combustion, we are disrupting the flows of elements through
the soils, oceans, biota, and atmosphere; we are changing the

biological and geological faces of the earth; we are influencing the climate; and we are driving plant and animal species out of existence at an accelerating rate. Humans now create entirely new elements and compounds; following recent breakthroughs in genetic engineering, they also have the capacity to create new infectious agents.

Many environmental alterations have helped to create comfortable and life-prolonging habitats. But humans have neither mastered nor come to a full understanding of the forces of nature, and many inventions and interventions are tried out without adequate concern for their possible consequences. Some have provoked terrible backlashes. As René Dubos observes, man "introduces new forces at such a rapid rate, and on such a wide scale, that the effects are upon him before he has a chance to evaluate their consequences."[17]

The surest way to avoid vicious environmental repercussions is to slow down the pace at which the ecosystem is being altered, and to keep human interventions within the boundaries of human understanding. But whether or not such a prudent course is adopted, humanity's impact on the environment—and hence ultimately on human well-being—has reached the point at which the close surveillance of the earth's life-support systems is essential.[18] Oceans, soils, the air, plants, and animals must be watched for signs of life-threatening changes—for the presence of unexpected pollutants and for unexpected effects from familiar substances or activities. Human populations must be scrutinized for telltale changes in the incidence of cancer or other environmentally induced diseases. Close tabs must also be kept on the number of birth defects, which signal threats to our genetic heritage.

Concern for human health leads inescapably to concern about humans' treatment of the natural environment—living and nonliving. But it also leads to concern about humans' treatment of one another; for the forces that promote poverty remain the greatest threats to human health.

Notes

Chapter 2. The Picture of Health Today

1. Unless otherwise noted, all data on life expectancy in this chapter are from Population Reference Bureau, *World Population Growth and Response, 1965–1975—A Decade of Global Action* (Washington, D.C.: April 1976). Throughout the chapter I have also drawn heavily on the excellent chapter on mortality trends and causes in United Nations, Department of Economic and Social Affairs, *The Determinants and Consequences of Population Trends,* Vol. 1 (New York: 1973). Throughout this chapter I have not listed sources for assertions or facts that are presented in more detail elsewhere in this book.
2. Leon F. Bouvier and Jean van der Tak, "Infant Mortality—Progress and Problems," *Population Bulletin,* April 1976; and Population Reference Bureau, "1976 World Population Data Sheet," Washington, D. C., 1976.
3. Alan Berg, *The Nutrition Factor* (Washington, D.C.: Brookings Institution, 1973); John Bryant, *Health and the Developing World* (Ithaca: Cornell University Press, 1969).
4. United Nations, Department of Economic and Social Affairs, *Poverty, Unemployment and Development Policy: A Case Study of Selected Issues with Reference to Kerala* (New York: 1975).
5. Victor R. Fuchs, *Who Shall Live? Health, Economics, and Social Choice* (New York: Basic Books, 1974), discusses some of the mortality-rate variations among subgroups within the United States. On Seventh-Day Adventists, see Marion M. Kristein, Charles B. Arnold, and Ernst L. Wynder, "Health, Economics and Preventive Care," *Science,* February 4, 1977.
6. United Nations, *The Determinants and Consequences of Population Trends.*
7. "Mortality Trends and Prospects," *WHO Chronicle,* December 1974.
8. Three good treatments of the factors contributing to recent mortality declines are: Carl E. Taylor and Marie-Françoise Hall, "Health, Population, and Economic Development," *Science,* August 11, 1967; M. J. Sharpston, "A Health Policy for Developing Countries," in Gerald Meier, ed., *Leading Issues in Economic Development,* 3rd ed. (New

York: Oxford University Press, 1976); and United Nations, *The Determi-nants and Consequences of Population Trends*, pp. 152–55. George J. Stolnitz argues that medical technologies have been the major factor in "International Mortality Trends: Some Main Facts and Implications," in United Nations, Department of Economic and Social Affairs, *The Popu-lation Debate: Dimensions and Perspectives*, Papers of the World Popu-lation Conference, Vol. 1 (New York: 1975).

Three classic articles on the causes of the modern decline in mortal-ity in Europe are Thomas McKeown and R. G. Brown, "Medical Evi-dence Related to English Population Changes in the Eighteenth Cen-tury," *Population Studies*, November 1955; Thomas McKeown and R. G. Record, "Reasons for the Decline of Mortality in England and Wales during the Nineteenth Century," *Population Studies*, November 1962; and Thomas McKeown, R. G. Brown, and R. G. Record, "An Interpreta-tion of the Modern Rise of Population in Europe," *Population Studies*, November 1972. Thomas McKeown's historical studies have culminated in his recent book, *The Modern Rise of Population* (New York: Aca-demic Press, 1976).

9. The report is summarized in "Mortality and Morbidity Trends, 1969–1972," *WHO Chronicle*, August 1975.

10. Michael Sharpston, *Factors Determining the Health Situation in Devel-oping Countries* (Washington, D.C.: World Bank Staff Working Paper, draft, 1974–75).

11. *Ibid.*

12. World Health Organization, "Community Water Supply and Wastewa-ter Disposal (Mid-Decade Progress Report)," Report by the Director-General, Geneva, May 6, 1976. See also C.S. Pineo and D. V. Subrah-manyam, "Community Water Supply and Excreta Disposal Situation in the Developing Countries: A Commentary," World Health Organiza-tion, Geneva, 1975; and World Bank, *Village Water Supply*, March 1976.

13. R. E. Novick, "Basic Sanitary Services: Water Supply—Excreta, Sewage and Solid Waste Disposal—Drainage," World Health Organization, Ge-neva, 1976.

14. Novick, "Basic Sanitary Services"; World Health Organization, "Com-munity Water Supply and Wastewater Disposal."

15. Donald A. Henderson, "The Eradication of Smallpox," *Scientific Ameri-can*, October 1976. The smallpox virus will be preserved in selected laboratories.

16. Richard W. Goodgame and William B. Greenough III, "Cholera in Africa: A Message for the West," *Annals of Internal Medicine*, January 1975; U. S. Agency for International Development, *Interim Report of the Task Force on Cholera* (Washington, D. C.: June 17, 1971).

17. World Health Organization, "Tropical Diseases Today—The Challenge and the Opportunity," Geneva, August 1975; "Epitaph for Global Ma-laria Eradication?" *Lancet*, July 5, 1975; *WHO Expert Committee on Malaria*, Sixteenth Report (Geneva: 1974).

18. World Health Organization, "Tropical Diseases Today"; *Disposal of Community Wastewater*, Report of a WHO Expert Committee (Ge-neva: 1974).

19. World Health Organization, "Tropical Diseases Today"; and World

Health Organization, "A Special Programme for Research and Training in Tropical Diseases—the Diseases," Geneva, September 1975.

20. Wilson G. Smillie, "Public Health in the United States—The Beginnings," in Edwin D. Kilbourne and Wilson G. Smillie, eds., *Human Ecology and Public Health*, Fourth Edition (London: Collier-MacMillan, 1969).

21. United Nations, *The Determinants and Consequences of Population Trends.*

22. *Ibid.* Age distribution of coronary deaths calculated for France, United Kingdom, Japan, and United States from *World Health Statistics Annual, 1972* (Geneva: World Health Organization, 1975).

23. Age distribution of cancer deaths calculated for France, United Kingdom, Japan, and United States from *World Health Statistics Annual, 1972.*

24. Environment Agency, *Quality of the Environment in Japan—1972* (Tokyo: 1972).

25. Jun Ui, ed., *Polluted Japan: Reports by Members of the Jishu-Koza Citizen's Movement* (Tokyo: Jishu-Koza, 1972); W. Eugene Smith and Aileen M. Smith, *Minamata* (New York: Holt, Rinehart and Winston, 1975); Environment Agency, "Pollution Related Measures and Relief Measures in Japan," Tokyo, May 1972; Norrie Huddle and Michael Reich with Nahrum Stiskin, *Island of Dreams* (New York: Autumn Press, 1975).

26. See U.S. House of Representatives, Committee on Science and Technology, *The Costs and Effects of Chronic Exposure to Low-Level Pollutants in the Environment*, Hearings, November 7–17, 1975. An important review of mutagenic risks and screening needs is "Environmental Mutagenic Hazards," *Science*, February 14, 1975.

Chapter 3. The Human Geography of Undernutrition

1. The latest recommended nutritional requirements are in *Energy and Protein Requirements: Report of a Joint FAO/WHO Ad Hoc Expert Committee* (Rome: Food and Agriculture Organization and World Health Organization, 1973). Nevin S. Scrimshaw, "An Analysis of Past and Present Recommended Dietary Allowances for Protein in Health and Disease," *New England Journal of Medicine*, January 15 and January 27, 1976; and C. Garza, *et al.*, "Human Protein Requirements: The Effect of Variations of Energy Intake Within the Maintenance Range," *American Journal of Clinical Nutrition*, March 1976, both suggest the inadequacy of current protein standards. In *Man Adapting* (New Haven: Yale University Press, 1965), pp. 81–85, René Dubos discusses nutritional adaptation.

2. Thomas T. Poleman, "World Food: A Perspective," *Science*, May 9, 1975, critically reviews past global nutrition surveys. The U.N. estimates are in United Nations, *Assessment of the World Food Situation, Present and Future* (Rome: U. N. World Food Conference, November 1974). The World Bank has recently reviewed the extent of undernutrition in Shlomo Reutlinger and Marcelo Selowsky, *Malnu-*

trition and Poverty: Magnitude and Policy Options (Washington, D. C.: 1976).

3. Derrick B. Jelliffe, "Tropical Problems in Nutrition," *Annals of Internal Medicine*, Vol. 79, 1973, p. 701.

4. Jelliffe, "Tropical Problems in Nutrition"; Moisés Béhar, "Poverty Must Take the Blame," *People* (London), Vol. 3, No. 1, 1976. By the commonly used Gomez system of classification, the mildly undernourished weigh 75–90 percent, the moderately undernourished weigh 60–75 percent, and the severely undernourished less than 60 percent of their expected weights according to age.

5. J. J. Bengoa, "The State of World Nutrition," World Health Organization, Geneva, 1973; W. R. Aykroyd, *Conquest of Deficiency Diseases* (Geneva: World Health Organization, 1970); Alfred Sommer, "Xerophthalmia: A Status Report," *Tropical Doctor*, April 1976.

6. UNICEF survey not available for citation. Other useful reviews of India's nutrition situation that reach similar conclusions are Davidson R. Gwatkin, *Health and Nutrition in India* (New Delhi: Ford Foundation, January 1974); C. Gopalan, *et al.*, *Diet Atlas of India* (Hyderabad: National Institute of Nutrition, 1971); and C. Gopalan and K. V. Raghavan, *Nutrition Atlas of India* (Hyderabad: National Institute of Nutrition, 1971).

7. Thomas Stapleton, "Child Health in China," *Journal of Tropical Pediatrics and Environmental Child Health*, September 1973; Jay M. Arena, "Nutritional Status of China's Children: An Overview," *Nutrition Reviews*, October 1974.

8. K. V. Bailey, "Malnutrition in the African Region," *WHO Chronicle*, Vol. 29, 1975, p. 354; "Tackling Nutrition Problems in Africa," *WHO Chronicle*, Vol. 30, 1976, p. 28.

9. Pan American Health Organization, "Food and Nutrition Situation in the Latin American and Caribbean Countries," in *Final Report of the 23rd Meeting of the Directing Council of PAHO* (Washington, D. C.: October 1975); Jelliffe, "Tropical Problems in Nutrition."

10. Freeman H. Quimby, "Hunger and Malnutrition in the United States: How Much?" Congressional Research Service, Library of Congress, Washington, D.C., May 1, 1975; Department of Health, Education and Welfare, *Preliminary Findings of the First Health and Nutrition Examination Survey, U. S., 1971–72: Dietary Intake and Biochemical Findings* (Washington, D.C.: G.P.O., January 1974), and *Anthropometric and Clinical Findings* (Washington, D.C.: G.P.O., April 1975).

11. Ruth Rice Puffer and Carlos V. Serrano, *Patterns of Mortality in Childhood* (Washington, D. C.: Pan American Health Organization, 1973).

12. *Ibid.*

13. David Morley, *Paediatric Priorities in the Developing World* (London: Butterworths, 1973); Herbert G. Birch, "Malnutrition, Learning, and Intelligence," *American Journal of Public Health*, Vol. 62, No. 6, 1972.

14. Leonardo J. Mata, *et al.*, "Influence of Recurrent Infections on Nutrition and Growth of Children in Guatemala," *American Journal of Clinical Nutrition*, November 1972; Gerald T. Keusch, "Malnutrition and Infection: Deadly Allies," *Natural History*, November 1975.

15. Keusch, "Malnutrition and Infection."
16. Michael C. Latham, "Nutrition and Infection in National Develop-
    ment," *Science,* May 9, 1975; Morley, *Paediatric Priorities.*
17. Nevin S. Scrimshaw and Moisés Béhar, "Protein Malnutrition in Young
    Children," *Science,* June 30, 1961.
18. Nevin S. Scrimshaw, Carl E. Taylor, and John E. Gordon, *Interactions
    of Nutrition and Infection* (Geneva: World Health Organization, 1968).
19. Derrick B. Jelliffe and E. F. Patrice Jelliffe, "Human Milk, Nutrition, and
    the World Resource Crisis," *Science,* May 9, 1975; Alan Berg, *The Nutri-
    tion Factor* (Washington, D. C.: Brookings Institution, 1973); Jon E.
    Rohde, "Human Milk in the Second Year: Nutritional and Economic
    Considerations for Indonesia," *Paediatrica Indonesiana,* November-
    December 1974; Ted Greiner, *The Promotion of Bottle Feeding by
    Multinational Corporations: How Advertising and the Health Profes-
    sions Have Contributed* (Ithaca, New York: Cornell International Nutri-
    tion Monograph Series No. 2, 1975).
20. Scrimshaw, Taylor, and Gordon, *Interactions of Nutrition and Infection.*
21. National Academy of Sciences, "The Relationship of Nutrition to Brain
    Development and Behavior," Washington, D. C., June 1973. For an
    excellent, up-to-date review of the problem see Myron Winick, *Malnu-
    trition and Brain Development* (New York: Oxford University Press,
    1976).
22. Joaquín Cravioto and Elsa DeLicardie, "Environmental Correlates of
    Severe Clinical Malnutrition and Language Development in Survivors
    from Kwashiorkor or Marasmus," in *Nutrition, the Nervous System, and
    Behavior* (Washington, D. C.: Pan American Health Organization,
    1972); "Mental Retardation from Malnutrition: 'Irreversible'," *Journal
    of the American Medical Association,* September 30, 1968.
23. Pek Hien Liang, *et al.,* "Evaluation of Mental Development in Relation
    to Early Malnutrition," *American Journal of Clinical Nutrition,* De-
    cember 1967. In "Malnutrition, Learning, and Intelligence," Birch re-
    views numerous studies of undernutrition and intelligence.
24. Roger Lewin, "The Poverty of Undernourished Brains," *New Scientist,*
    October 24, 1974; John Dobbing, "Lasting Deficits and Distortions of the
    Adult Brain Following Infantile Undernutrition," in *Nutrition, the Ner-
    vous System, and Behavior.*
25. Myron Winick, *et al.,* "Malnutrition and Environmental Enrichment by
    Early Adoption," *Science,* December 19, 1975.
26. National Academy of Sciences, *The Relationship of Nutrition to Brain
    Development and Behavior;* Roger Lewin, "Starved Brains," *Psychol-
    ogy Today,* September 1975. "Malnutrition and Mental Development,"
    WHO Chronicle, Vol. 28, 1974, p. 101, stresses the lack of strong proof
    that mild undernutrition impairs mental development.
27. Michael C. Latham and Francisco Cobos, "The Effects of Malnutrition
    on Intellectual Development and Learning," *American Journal of Pub-
    lic Health,* July 1971; Berg, *The Nutrition Factor.*
28. "Tackling Nutrition Problems in Africa," *WHO Chronicle,* Vol. 30, 1976,
    p. 29.
29. Berg, *The Nutrition Factor.* On the advantages of breast feeding see also
    Jelliffe, "Human Milk, Nutrition, and the World Resource Crisis"; and
    Rohde, "Human Milk in the Second Year."

30. Michael C. Latham, "Introduction," in Greiner, *The Promotion of Bottle Feeding by Multinational Corporations*. See also Ted Greiner, *Regulation and Education: Strategies for Solving the Bottle Feeding Problem* (Ithaca, New York: Cornell International Nutrition Monograph Series No. 4, 1977), for a useful review of possible actions to control the spread of bottle feeding.

Chapter 4. *Mutinous Bounty: Hazards of the Affluent Diet*

1. Jean Mayer, "The Bitter Truth About Sugar," *New York Times Magazine*, June 20, 1976.
2. M. E. Moore, *et al.*, "Obesity, Social Class and Mental Illness," *Journal of the American Medical Association*, Vol. 181, 1962, p. 138; Jean Mayer, ed., *U. S. Nutrition Policies in the Seventies* (San Francisco: Freeman and Co., 1973).
3. R. S. Goodhart, ed., *Modern Nutrition in Health and Disease* (Philadelphia: Lea and Febiger, 1973); "Overweight: Its Prevention and Significance," reprints from *Statistical Bulletin*, Metropolitan Life Insurance Company, New York, 1960; "Statement of Dr. Theodore Cooper," in U. S. Senate, Select Committee on Nutrition and Human Needs, *Diet Related to Killer Diseases*, Hearings, July 27–28, 1976.
4. R. K. Oates, "Infant Feeding Practices," *British Medical Journal*, 1973 (Vol. 2), p. 762.
5. Jean Mayer, "Hidden Bonds: Obesity, Heredity, and Hunger," *World Health*, February 1974.
6. Eunice Tsomondo and Jim Jones, "Obesity: A Disease of Indolence and Affluence," *Central African Journal of Medicine*, January 1974.
7. Mayer, "Hidden Bonds."
8. Lars Werko, "Can We Prevent Heart Disease?", *Annals of Internal Medicine*, February 1971; Department of Health, Education, and Welfare, *Monthly Vital Statistics Report*, May 1975; "Special Communication," *Journal of the American Medical Association*, March 4, 1974.
9. S. G. Sarvotham and J. N. Berry, "Prevalence of Coronary Heart Disease in an Urban Population in Northern India," *Circulation*, June 1968; "Heart Disease Problems in China," *Annals of Internal Medicine*, January 1974; World Health Organization, *Second Regional Seminar on Cardiovascular Diseases* (Manila: 1975).
10. W. B. Kannel, *et al.*, "Factors of Risk in the Development of Coronary Heart Disease: Six Year Follow-up Experience: The Framingham Study," *Annals of Internal Medicine*, Vol. 55, No. 33, 1961; American Heart Association, "Heart Facts," New York, 1973.
11. E. Personen, *et al.*, "Thickenings in the Coronary Arteries in Infancy as an Indication of Genetic Factor in Coronary Heart Disease," *Circulation*, February 1975. An interesting community program in Finland designed to prevent cardiovascular diseases is described in Pekka Puska, "High-Risk Hearts," *World Health*, October 1976.
12. Kannel, "Factors of Risk"; Committee on Nutrition, "Childhood Diet and Coronary Heart Disease," *Pediatrics*, February 1972.

13. Food and Nutrition Board of the National Academy of Sciences and Council on Food and Nutrition of the American Medical Association, "Diet and Coronary Heart Disease," Washington, D.C., July 1972. For a useful review of dietary influences on coronary diseases see William E. Connor and Sonja L. Connor, "The Key Role of Nutritional Factors in the Prevention of Coronary Heart Disease," *Preventive Medicine,* Vol. 1, 1972, p. 49.

14. H. I. Russek, "Behaviour Patterns, Stress, and Coronary Heart Disease," *American Family Physician,* April 1974.

15. National Board of Health and Welfare, *Diet and Health* (Stockholm: 1972); R. A. Shorey, *et al.,* "Efficacy of Diet and Exercise in the Reduction of Serum Cholesterol and Triglycerides in Free-Living Adult Males," *American Journal of Clinical Nutrition,* May 1976; Department of Health and Social Security, *Diet and Coronary Heart Disease* (London: Her Majesty's Stationary Office, 1974).

16. American Heart Association, "Diet and Coronary Heart Disease," New York, 1973; R. M. Feeley, *et al.,* "Cholesterol Content of Foods," *Journal of the American Dietetic Association,* Vol. 61, 1972, p. 134.

17. "Assessment of the State of Nutrition Science," *Nutrition Today,* January/February 1977.

18. Ray Gifford, Jr., "Hypertension 1975," *Drug Therapy,* May 1975; American Heart Association, "Heart Facts."

19. Lewis K. Dahl, "Salt and Hypertension," *American Journal of Clinical Nutrition,* February 1972; L. C. Isaacson, "Sodium Intake and Hypertension," *Lancet,* 1963 (Vol. 1), p. 946; A. G. Shaper, "Cardiovascular Disease in the Tropics," *British Medical Journal,* September 30, 1972.

20. R. L. Weinsier, "Overview: Salt and the Development of Essential Hypertension," *Preventive Medicine,* March 1976.

21. "More Proof of Salt-Hypertension Link," *Journal of the American Medical Association,* March 28, 1977. Naosuke Sasaki, "High Blood Pressure and the Salt Intake of the Japanese," *Japanese Heart Journal,* July 1962.

22. E. Harburg, *et al.,* "Socio-Ecological Stress, Suppressed Hostility, Skin Color, and Black-White Male Blood Pressure: Detroit," *Psychosomatic Medicine,* July-August 1973; Joseph Eyer, "Hypertension as a Disease of Modern Society," *International Journal of Health Services,* Vol. 5, No. 4, 1975.

23. W. E. Morton, "Hypertension and Drinking Water Constituents in Colorado," *American Journal of Public Health,* July 1971.

24. U. S. Senate, Select Committee on Nutrition and Human Needs, *Nutrition and Diseases—1974,* Part 4, Hearings, February 26, 1974; *Report of the National Commission on Diabetes to the Congress of the United States,* Vol. 1 (Washington, D. C.: National Institutes of Health, 1975). Methods of recording diabetes-related deaths have changed over time, but the increase in diabetes incidence is genuine nonetheless.

25. R. V. Sattre, "The Problem of Diabetes Mellitus in India," *Journal of the Indian Medical Association,* July 1, 1973; M. Sankale, "Les Particularités du Diabetes Sucre chez le Noir Africain," *Journées de Diabetologie de l'Hotel Dieu,* May 1971.

26. N. Kuzuye and K. Kosaka, "Diabetics in Japan," in *Symposium on Diabetes in Asian People,* Proceedings of the 13th Annual Meeting of the Japanese Diabetic Society, Kumomoto, May 22, 1970.

27. D. Rimoin, "Inheritance in Diabetes Mellitus," *Medical Clinics of North America,* July 1971; U.S. Senate, *Nutrition and Diseases—1974;* "Statement of Dr. Theodore Cooper." Articles suggesting a link between high sugar consumption and diabetes prevalence include G. D. Campbell, "Diabetes in Asians and Africans in and Around Durban," *South African Medical Journal,* November 30, 1963; and A. M. Cohen, *et al.,* "Genetics and Diet as Factors in the Development of Diabetes Mellitus," *Metabolism,* March 1972.

28. Denis P. Burkitt, "Some Neglected Leads to Cancer Causation," *Journal of the National Cancer Institute,* November 1971; D. P. Burkitt, A. R. P. Walker, and N. S. Painter, "Effect of Dietary Fibre on Stools and Transit-Time, and Its Role in the Causation of Disease," *Lancet,* December 30, 1972.

29. G. S. Drasar and Doreen Irving, "Environmental Factors and Cancer of the Colon and Breast," *British Journal of Cancer,* Vol. 27, 1973, p. 167; William Haenszel, *et al.,* "Large-Bowel Cancer in Hawaiian Japanese," *Journal of the National Cancer Institute,* December 1973.

30. M. J. Hill, "Colon Cancer: A Disease of Fibre Depletion or of Dietary Excess," *Digestion,* 1974 (Vol. 2) p. 289; Ernst L. Wynder, "The Epidemiology of Large Bowel Cancer," *Cancer Research,* November 1975.

31. John W. Berg, "Can Nutrition Explain the Pattern of International Epidemiology of Hormone-Dependent Cancers?" *Cancer Research,* November 1975; Ernst L. Wynder, "On the Key Importance of Nutrition in Cancer Causation and Prevention," presented to the American Cancer Society's Sixteenth Science Writers Seminar, St. Augustine, Florida, March 22–27, 1974.

32. Ernst L. Wynder, "Nutrition and Cancer," *Federation Proceedings,* May 1, 1976; D. Mark Hegsted, "Summary of the Conference on Nutrition in the Causation of Cancer," *Cancer Research,* November 1975.

33. "Food and Nutrition Policies," *British Medical Journal,* August 21, 1976; Colin Blythe, "Eating Our Way Out of Debt and Disease," *New Scientist,* May 6, 1976; Colin Blythe, "Problems of Diet and Affluence," *Food Policy,* February 1976; U. S. Senate, Select Committee on Nutrition and Human Needs, *Nutrition and Health II,* Committee Print, July 1976; and "Nutrition, Health, and Public Policy," Statement of Dr. Beverly Winikoff, in U. S. Senate, Select Committee on Nutrition and Human Needs, *Diet Related to Killer Diseases,* Hearings, July 27–28, 1976, all discuss the case for national nutrition strategies in developed countries.

34. G. T. T. Molitor, "Anticipating Public Policy Issues: Nutrition, Diet, Health, and Food Quality," U. S. General Accounting Office, Washington, D. C., July 1976; National Board of Health and Welfare, *Diet and Exercise* (Stockholm: 1972); Royal Norwegian Ministry of Agriculture, "Report to the Storting No. 32 (1975–76) on Norwegian Nutrition and Food Policy," Oslo, November 7, 1975; "Dietary Goals for the United States," prepared by the staff of the Select Committee on Nutrition and Human Needs, U. S. Senate, January 1977.

35. Hegsted, "Summary of the Conference on Nutrition in the Causation of Cancer."

Chapter 5. Cancer: A Social Disease

1. Ernst L. Wynder and Gio B. Gori, "Contribution of the Environment to Cancer Incidence: An Epidemiologic Exercise," *Journal of the National Cancer Institute,* April 1977. Quote from Umberto Saffiotti, "Prevention of Occupational Cancer—Toward an Integrated Program of Governmental Action: Role of the National Cancer Institute," presented to the Conference on Occupational Carcinogenesis, *Annals of the New York Academy of Sciences,* May 28, 1976.
2. Russell E. Train, "Testing Chemicals, Not People: Bringing the Chemical Threat Under Control," presented to National Press Club, Washington, D.C., February 26, 1976; Irving J. Selikoff, "Persistence of Carcinogenic Agents in Tissues," presented to the American Cancer Society's Eighteenth Science Writers' Seminar, St. Petersburg Beach, Florida, March 26–30, 1976.
3. Thomas H. Maugh II and Jean L. Marx, *Seeds of Destruction: The "Science" Report on Cancer Research* (New York: Plenum Press, 1975).
4. John Cairns, "The Cancer Problem," *Scientific American,* November 1975; Sir Richard Doll, "Strategy for Detection of Cancer Hazards to Man," *Nature,* February 17, 1977.
5. "Developments in the Work of the IARC," *WHO Chronicle,* Vol. 30, 1976, p. 194.
6. Kenneth J. Rothman, "Alcohol," in Joseph F. Fraumeni, Jr., ed., *Persons at High Risk of Cancer* (New York: Academic Press, 1975).
7. W. C. Hueper, "Public Health Hazards from Environmental Chemical Carcinogens, Mutagens and Teratogens," *Health Physics,* November 1971; Cairns, "The Cancer Problem"; Umberto Saffiotti, "Comments on the Scientific Basis for the Delaney Clause," *Preventive Medicine,* March 1973.
8. Benjamin F. Byrd, "The President's Report," presented to the American Cancer Society's Eighteenth Science Writers' Seminar, St. Petersburg Beach, Florida, March 26–30, 1976; American Cancer Society, "Cancer and the Environment," New York, February 13, 1976.
9. Ernst L. Wynder, "Introductory Remarks," *Cancer Research,* November 1975.
10. John W. Berg, "Diet," in Fraumeni, *Persons at High Risk of Cancer.*
11. Pelayo Correa, *et al.,* "A Model for Gastric Cancer Epidemiology," *Lancet,* July 12, 1975; John H. Weisburger and Ronald Raineri, "Dietary Factors and the Etiology of Gastric Cancer," *Cancer Research,* November 1975; Robert Zaldivar and Harry Robinson, "Epidemiological Investigation on Stomach Cancer Mortality in Chileans: Association with Nitrate Fertilizer," *Zeitschrift für Krebsforschung,* Vol. 80, 1973, p. 289; M. J. Hill, G. Hawksworth, and G. Tattersall, "Bacteria, Nitrosamines and Cancer of the Stomach," *British Journal of Cancer,* Vol. 28, 1973, p. 562; William Lijinsky, "Health Problems Associated with Nitrites and Nitrosamines," *Ambio,* Vol. 5, No. 1, 1976.
12. H. Hormozdiari, *et al.,* "Dietary Factors and Esophageal Cancer in the Caspian Littoral of Iran," *Cancer Research,* November 1975.
13. Paula Cook, "Cancer of the Esophagus in Africa," *British Journal of Cancer,* Vol. 25, 1971, p. 853; "Oesophageal Carcinoma in Africa," *Lancet,* March 18, 1972.

14. Kenneth J. Rothman, "Alcohol," in Fraumeni, *Persons at High Risk of Cancer;* International Agency for Research on Cancer, *Annual Report 1975* (Lyon, France: 1975).
15. Rothman, "Alcohol."
16. "Cancer and Food," *Lancet,* November 17, 1973; Berg, "Diet"; International Agency for Research on Cancer, *Annual Report 1975.*
17. Seymour Jablon, "Radiation," in Fraumeni, *Persons At High Risk of Cancer.*
18. N. T. Racoveanu, "Geographic Distribution of Cancer in Middle East Countries," World Health Organization, Alexandria, Egypt, n.d.
19. Arthur C. Upton, "Physical Carcinogenesis: Radiation—History and Sources," in F. F. Becker, ed., *Cancer, Vol. 1* (New York: Plenum, 1975); John T. Edsall, "Toxicity of Plutonium and Some of the Actinides," *Bulletin of the Atomic Scientists,* September 1976.
20. National Academy of Sciences, *The Effects on Populations of Exposure to Low Levels of Ionizing Radiation* (Washington, D.C.: November 1972); "Thresholds and Low-level Irradiation Effects," *Lancet,* September 15, 1973.
21. Doll, "Strategy for Detection of Cancer Hazards to Man"; Barbara J. Culliton, "Breast Cancer: Second Thoughts About Routine Mammography," *Science,* August 13, 1976.
22. *Environmental Change and Resulting Impacts on Health* (Geneva: World Health Organization Technical Report Series No. 292, 1964); Claire Nader, "The Dispute Over Safe Uses of X rays in Medical Practice," *Health Physics,* July 1975; World Health Organization, Regional Office for the Western Pacific, "Twenty-Fifth Annual Report of the Regional Director to the Regional Committee for the Western Pacific," Manila, June 1975.
23. J. Martin Brown, "Health, Safety, and Social Issues," in W. C. Reynolds, ed., *The California Nuclear Initiative* (Palo Alto: Stanford University Institute for Energy Studies, April 1976), provides an excellent discussion of potential health hazards from routine nuclear power operations. See also W. H. M. Ellett and A. C. B. Richardson, "Estimates of the Cancer Risk Due to Nuclear Electric Power Generation," Environmental Protection Agency, Washington, D. C., October 1976.
24. Denis Hayes, *Rays of Hope* (New York: W. W. Norton, 1977).
25. Hayes, *Rays of Hope;* Amory Lovins, "Energy Strategy: The Road Not Taken?" *Foreign Affairs,* October 1976.
26. Arthur Kallet and F. J. Schlink, *100,000,000 Guinea Pigs: Dangers in Everyday Foods, Drugs, and Cosmetics* (New York: Vanguard Press, 1932).
27. Robert Hoover and Joseph F. Fraumeni, Jr., "Drugs," in Fraumeni, *Persons at High Risk of Cancer;* Kenneth L. Noller, "DES and Pregnancy: Lower Reproductive Tract Changes in Offspring," *BioScience,* September 1976. Those eating beef liver in the United States may consume slight traces of DES, which is used as a growth stimulant in cattle production. Efforts to ban this use of the hormone are now enmeshed in legal disputes.
28. Train, "Testing Chemicals, Not People."
29. For example, see S. A. Hall, "Environmental Risks from Chemical Carcinogens in East Africa," in Peter Clifford, C. Allen Linsell, and Geoffrey

L. Timms, eds., *Cancer in Africa* (Nairobi: East African Publishing House, 1968).

30. Gina Bari Koluta, "Chemical Carcinogens: Industry Adopts Controversial 'Quick' Tests," *Science,* June 18, 1976, discusses the potential uses of bacterial tests.

31. "Evaluation of Environmental Carcinogens," Report to the Surgeon General by the Ad Hoc Committee on the Evaluation of Low Levels of Environmental Chemical Carcinogens, April 22, 1970, reprinted by National Institutes of Health, Bethesda, Maryland. Problems in the testing and control of carcinogens are also discussed in Samuel J. Epstein, "Environmental Determinants of Human Cancer," *Cancer Research,* October 1974.

32. John Higginson, "A Hazardous Society? Individual Versus Community Responsibility in Cancer Prevention," *American Journal of Public Health,* April 1976.

33. Cairns, "The Cancer Problem."

Chapter 6. The Unnatural History of Tobacco

1. Bernardino Ramazzini, *Diseases of Workers,* translated by Wilmer Cave Wright (New York: Hafner Publishing Co., 1964).

2. Edmund Smith, ed., *A Counter-Blaste to Tobacco (Written by King James I)* (Edinburgh: E. and G. Goldsmid, 1885).

3. D. D. Reid, "The Beginnings of Bronchitis," *Proceedings of the Royal Society of Medicine,* April 1969.

4. Joseph Knight, ed., *Pipe and Pouch: The Smoker's Own Book of Poetry* (Boston: Joseph Knight Co., 1895); Ramazzini, *Diseases of Workers.*

5. John Nance, *The Gentle Tasaday* (New York: Harcourt Brace Jovanovich, 1975).

6. George Louis Beer, *The Origins of the British Colonial System, 1578–1660* (New York: Macmillan, 1922).

7. Peter Osnos, "Soviet Anti-Smoking Campaign Fails," *Washington Post,* October 17, 1976.

8. Among the pioneering studies on smoking, lung cancer, and death rates were Richard Doll and A. Bradford Hill, "Smoking and Carcinoma of the Lung," *British Medical Journal,* September 30, 1950; Ernst L. Wynder and Evards A. Graham, "Tobacco Smoking as a Possible Etiologic Factor in Bronchiogenic Carcinoma," *Journal of the American Medical Association,* May 27, 1950; E. Cuyler Hammond and Daniel Horn, "The Relationship Between Human Smoking Habits and Death Rates," *Journal of the American Medical Association,* August 7, 1954; Editorial, "Cancer of the Lung," *New England Journal of Medicine,* Vol. 249, 1953, p. 465.

9. *Smoking and Health,* Summary and Report of the Royal College of Physicians of London on Smoking in Relation to Cancer of the Lung and Other Diseases (London: Pitman Medical Publishing Co., 1962); *Smoking and Health,* Report of the Advisory Committee to the Surgeon General of the Public Health Service (Princeton: D. Van Nostrand Co., 1964).

10. *Smoking and Health,* Report of the Advisory Committee to the Surgeon General; E. Cuyler Hammond, "Multiple Factor Etiology in Cancer," presentation to the American Cancer Society's Eighteenth Science Writers' Seminar, St. Petersburg Beach, Florida, March 26–30, 1976; Gio B. Gori, "Statement Before the Select Committee on Nutrition and Human Needs, U. S. Senate," July 28, 1976.
11. Benjamin F. Byrd, "The President's Report," presented to the American Cancer Society's Eighteenth Science Writers' Seminar, St. Petersburg Beach, Florida, March 26–30, 1976.
12. American Heart Association, "Heart Facts," New York, 1973.
13. E. W. Anderson, *et al.,* "Effect of Low-Level Carbon Monoxide Exposure on Onset and Duration of Angina Pectoris," *Annals of Internal Medicine,* Vol. 79, 1973, p. 46; S. M. Ayres and M. E. Buehler, "The Effects of Urban Air Pollution on Health," *Clinical Pharmacology and Therapeutics,* Vol. 11, No. 3, 1970; W. B. Kannel and W. P. Castelli, "Significance of Nicotine, Carbon Monoxide and other Smoke Components in the Development of Cardiovascular Disease," in Ernst L. Wynder, *et al.,* eds., *Smoking and Health. I. Modifying the Risk for the Smoker.* Proceedings of the 3rd World Conference on Smoking and Health, 1975 (Washington, D.C.: U.S. Department of Health, Education, and Welfare, 1976); U.S. Department of Health, Education, and Welfare, Public Health Service, "The Health Consequences of Smoking, 1975," Atlanta, June 1975.
14. *Smoking and Health,* Report of the Advisory Committee to the Surgeon General.
15. M. A. Russell, P. V. Cole, and E. Brown, "Absorption by Non-Smokers of Carbon Monoxide from Air Polluted by Tobacco Smoke," *Lancet,* March 17, 1973; "Smoking and Disease: The Evidence Reviewed," *WHO Chronicle,* August 1975; *New York Times,* March 25, 1976.
16. David Rush and Edward H. Kass, "Maternal Smoking: A Reassessment of the Association with Perinatal Mortality," *American Journal of Epidemiology,* Vol. 96, No. 3, 1972; Mary B. Meyer, James A. Tonascia, and Carol Buck, "The Interrelationship of Maternal Smoking and Increased Perinatal Mortality with Other Risk Factors," *American Journal of Epidemiology,* Vol. 100, No. 6, 1975; Susan Harlap and A.M. Davies, "Infant Admissions to Hospital and Maternal Smoking," *Lancet,* March 30, 1974; "Smoking and Disease: The Evidence Reviewed."
17. U.S. Department of Health, Education, and Welfare, Public Health Service, "Adult Use of Tobacco—1975," Atlanta, June 1976.
18. U.S. Department of Health, Education, and Welfare, Public Health Service, *Health: United States, 1975* (Rockville, Md.: 1976); "Smoking and Disease: The Evidence Reviewed."
19. Cigarette consumption figures supplied by U.S. Department of Agriculture.
20. Daniel S. Joly, "Cigarette Smoking in Latin America: A Survey in Eight Cities," Pan American Health Organization, Washington, D.C., 1973.
21. R. N. Banerjee, "Prevalence of Habit-Forming Drugs and Smoking Among the College Students—A Survey," *Indian Medical Journal,* August 1963; O. P. Arya and F. J. Bennett, "Smoking Amongst University Students in Uganda," *East African Medical Journal,* January 1970.

22. Prof. D. Femi-Pearse, private communication, May 10, 1976.
23. Alan MacFarlane, *Resources and Population: A Study of the Gurungs of Nepal* (Cambridge: Cambridge University Press, 1976).
24. Thomas Whiteside, "Smoking Still," *New Yorker,* November 18, 1974.
25. Michael Pertschuk, "Smoking in China," *Washington Post,* October 17, 1976.
26. Tobacco Institute, "Some Facts About Tobacco," Washington, D. C., 1975; D. Femi-Pearse, A. Adeniyi-Jones, and A.B. Oke, "Respiratory Symptoms and Their Relationship to Cigarette Smoking, Dusty Occupations and Domestic Air Pollution," *West African Medical Journal,* June 1973.
27. Samuel S. Epstein, "The Political and Economic Basis of Cancer," *Technology Review,* July/August 1976.
28. Data on U.S. and European tobacco export-promotion activities, and on tobacco shipments under P.L. 480, supplied by U.S. Department of Agriculture.
29. James Fallows, "The Cigarette Scandal," *Washington Monthly,* February 1976.
30. M.A.H. Russell, "Realistic Goals for Smoking and Health," *Lancet,* February 16, 1974.
31. *New York Times,* March 9, 1975.
32. A WHO Expert Committee recommends a series of national and international policies to discourage smoking in "Smoking and Disease: The Evidence Reviewed." For the full report see *Smoking and Health,* Report of a WHO Expert Committee (Geneva: WHO Technical Report Series No. 568, 1975).
33. U.S. Department of Health, Education, and Welfare, Public Health Service, "Adult Use of Tobacco—1975."
34. Gio B. Gori, "Low-Risk Cigarettes: A Prescription," *Science,* December 17, 1976.
35. Daniel Horn, "Why People Smoke," *World Health,* December 1975.

Chapter 7. Something in the Air

1. E. C. Halliday, "A Historical Review of Atmospheric Pollution," in *Air Pollution* (Geneva: World Health Organization Monograph 46, 1961).
2. David A. Lynn, "Air Pollution," in W. W. Murdock, ed., *Environment: Resources, Pollution and Society,* 2nd ed. (Sunderland, Mass.: Sinauer Associates, 1975); National Academy of Sciences, *Air Quality and Automobile Emission Control, Vol. 1, Summary Report,* prepared for Committee on Public Works, September 1974 (Washington, D.C.: G.P.O., 1974).
3. Henry A. Schroeder, "A Sensible Look at Air Pollution by Metals," *Archives of Environmental Health,* December 1970; J. G. Thompson, *et al.,* "Asbestos as a Modern Urban Hazard," *South African Medical Journal,* January 19, 1963; E. P. Hardy, *et al.,* "Global Inventory and Distribution of Fallout Plutonium," *Nature,* Vol. 241, 1973, p. 444.
4. W. S. Cleveland, *et al.,* "Photochemical Air Pollution: Transport from the New York City area into Connecticut and Massachusetts," *Science,* January 19, 1976; *New York Times,* June 23, 1976.

5. *Ambio*, Vol. 5, Nos. 5–6, 1976; B. R. Ordonez, "Community Smelter Study in Ciudad Juarez, Mexico," mimeo (Mexico: Ministry of Health, n.d.).
6. Julian McCaull, "Discriminatory Air Pollution," *Environment*, March 1976.
7. L. P. Borkar, "Environmental Pollution with Particular Reference to Greater Bombay," and J. J. Deshpande, *et al.*, "Lead Content of Bombay, Calcutta and Delhi Air," *Indian Journal of Occupational Health*, May 1972.
8. L. Greenburg, *et al.*, "Report of an Air Pollution Incident in New York City, November 1953," *Public Health Reports*, January 1962; L. Greenburg, *et al.*, "Air Pollution, Influenza, and Mortality in New York City," *Archives of Environmental Health*, December 1967; *The Allegheny County Air Pollution Episode, November 16, 1975—November 20, 1975* (Philadelphia: Environmental Protection Agency, Region III, April 1976).
9. M. Glasser and L. Greenburg, "Air Pollution, Mortality, and Weather: New York City, 1960–64," *Archives of Environmental Health*, March 1971; H. Schimmel and L. Greenburg, "A Study of the Relation of Pollution to Mortality: New York City, 1963–1968," *Journal of the Air Pollution Control Association*, August 1972; A. C. Hexter and J. R. Goldsmith, "Carbon Monoxide: Association of Community Air Pollution with Mortality," *Science*, April 16, 1971.
10. I. T. T. Higgins, *Epidemiology of Chronic Respiratory Disease: A Literature Review*. (Washington, D. C.: Environmental Protection Agency, August 1974); W. W. Holland, *et al.*, "Respiratory Disease in England and the United States," *Archives of Environmental Health*, February 1965.
11. Higgins, *Epidemiology of Chronic Respiratory Disease*; Lung Program, National Heart and Lung Institute, *Respiratory Diseases: Task Force Report on Problems, Research Approaches, Needs* (Washington, D.C.: G.P.O., October 1972).
12. S. Ishikawa, *et al.*, "The 'Emphysema Profile' in Two Midwestern Cities in North America," *Archives of Environmental Health*, April 1969.
13. *Health Consequences of Sulfur Oxides: A Report from CHESS, 1970–71.* (Research Triangle Park, N.C.: National Environmental Research Center, May 1974).
14. W. W. Holland and D. D. Reid, "The Urban Factor in Chronic Bronchitis," *Lancet*, February 27, 1965.
15. H. P. Ribeiro, "Estudo das Correlações entre Infecções das Vias Aéreas Superiores, Bronquite Asmatiforme e Poluiçâo do Ar em Menores de 12 Anos em Santo André," *Pediatria Prática*, Vol. 42, April-May-June 1971; C. P. F. V. Murray, "La Contaminación Ambiental y la Salud del Niño," *Salud Publica de Mexico*, January-February 1973; E. G. Manzhenko, "The Effect of Air Pollution on the Health of the Juvenile Population," *Hygiene and Sanitation* (Moscow), Vol. 31, 1966, p. 107; *Health Consequences of Sulfur Oxides: A Report from CHESS, 1970–71;* J. W. B. Douglas and R. E. Waller, "Air Pollution and Respiratory Infection in Children," *British Journal of Preventive Social Medicine*, Vol. 20, 1966, p. 1; J. J. Collins, *et al.*, "Environmental Factors in Child Mortality in England and Wales," *American Journal of Epidemiology*, Vol. 93, No.

1, 1971; G. O. Sofoluwe, "Smoke Pollution in Dwellings of Infants with Bronchopneumonia," *Archives of Environmental Health,* May 1968; Jerald Bailey and Juan Correa, "Evaluation of the Profamilia Rural Family Planning Program," *Studies in Family Planning,* June 1975.

16. W. W. Holland, *et al.,* "Factors Influencing the Onset of Chronic Respiratory Disease," *British Medical Journal,* April 26, 1969; D. D. Reid, "The Beginnings of Bronchitis," *Proceedings of the Royal Society of Medicine,* April 1969.

17. E. W. Anderson, *et al.,* "Effect of Low-Level Carbon Monoxide Exposure on Onset and Duration of Angina Pectoris," *Annals of Internal Medicine,* Vol. 79, 1973, p. 46; S. M. Ayres and M. E. Buehler, "The Effects of Urban Air Pollution on Health," *Clinical Pharmacology and Therapeutics,* Vol. II, No. 3, 1970.

18. P. Buell and J. E. Dunn, "Relative Impact of Smoking and Air Pollution on Lung Cancer," *Archives of Environmental Health,* September 1967.

19. H. R. Menck, *et al.,* "Industrial Air Pollution: Possible Effect on Lung Cancer," *Science,* January 18, 1974.

20. W. Winkelstein, Jr. and S. Kantor, "Stomach Cancer," *Archives of Environmental Health,* April 1969; W. Winkelstein, Jr. and S. Kantor, "Prostatic Cancer: Relationship to Suspended Particulate Air Pollution," *American Journal of Public Health,* July 1969; D. Shapley, "Nitrosamines: Scientists on the Trail of Prime Suspect in Urban Cancer," *Science,* January 23, 1976.

21. W. J. Blot and J. F. Fraumeni, Jr., "Arsenical Air Pollution and Lung Cancer," *Lancet,* July 26, 1975.

22. John W. Gofman, "Estimated Production of Human Lung Cancers by Plutonium from Worldwide Fallout," (Dublin, California: Committee for Nuclear Responsibility, July 10, 1975).

23. John T. Edsall, "Toxicity of Plutonium and Some Other Actinides," *Bulletin of the Atomic Scientists,* September 1976.

24. M. B. McElroy, "Threats to the Atmosphere," *Harvard Magazine,* Vol. 78, No. 6, February 1976. National Academy of Sciences, *Halocarbons: Environmental Effects of Chlorofluoromethane Release* (Washington, D.C.: 1976).

25. National Academy of Sciences, *Air Quality and Automobile Emission Control Vol. I, Summary Report;* Lester Lave and Eugene Seskin, "Does Air Pollution Cause Mortality?" in *Statistics and the Environment,* Proceedings of the 4th Symposium, American Statistical Association, March 3–5, 1976, Washington, D.C.

26. Julian Gresser, "The 1973 Japanese Law for the Compensation of Pollution-Related Health Damage: An Introductory Assessment," *Environmental Law Reporter,* December 1975; Sydney Howe, "Making the Polluters Pay," *Washington Post,* January 30, 1977; Environment Agency, *Quality of the Environment in Japan—1975* (Tokyo: 1975).

27. Royal Commission on Environmental Pollution, *Fifth Report: Air Pollution Control: An Integrated Approach* (London: H.M. Stationary Office, January 1976).

28. Council of Environmental Quality, *Environmental Quality—1975* (Washington, D.C.: G.P.O., December 1975); Environment Agency, *Quality of the Environment in Japan—1975.*

29. Richard D. Stewart, *et al.,* "Carboxyhemoglobin Trend in Chicago

Blood Donors, 1970–1974," *Archives of Environmental Health*, November/December 1976.

30. Latin America's worsening air pollution problems are reviewed in *Pan American Air Pollution Monitoring Network, Report of Results, June 1967-December 1970* (Lima: Pan American Center for Sanitary Engineering and Environmental Sciences, 1971); Ricardo Haddad, "Contaminación del Aire," presented to PAHO Symposium on Environment, Health, and Development, Mexico City, July 29, 1974.

Chapter 8. Who Pays for Production?

1. Nicholas A. Ashford, *Crisis in the Workplace: Occupational Disease and Injury* (Cambridge, Mass.: MIT Press, 1976). Ashford's summary chapter is an excellent introduction to occupational health issues in developed countries.
2. Ashford, *Crisis in the Workplace.*
3. Brief reviews of major occupational hazards are included in World Health Organization, "Occupational Health Programme," Report by the Director General, Geneva, April 9, 1976; and Ashford, *Crisis in the Workplace.* In *Work Is Dangerous to Your Health* (New York: Vintage, 1973), Jeanne M. Stellman and Susan M. Daum review major U.S. occupational disease threats.
4. Samuel S. Epstein, "Cancer and the Environment: A Scientific Perspective," *I.U.D. Facts and Analysis*, No. 25 (A.F.L.–C.I.O.), February 1976.
5. Irving J. Selikoff, "Recent Perspectives in Occupational Cancer," *Ambio*, Vol. 4, No. 1, 1975; Irving J. Selikoff, "Household-Contact Asbestos: Neoplastic Risk," *Annals of the New York Academy of Sciences*, May 28, 1976; J. Wagner, *et al.*, "Epidemiology of Asbestos Cancers," *British Medical Bulletin*, Vol. 27, No. 1, 1971; *Wall Street Journal*, February 3, 1977; *Washington Post*, March 25, 1975.
6. William J. Blot and Joseph F. Fraumeni, Jr., "Arsenical Air Pollution and Lung Cancer," *Lancet*, July 26, 1975.
7. The Kepone story is drawn from newspaper accounts, principally in the *Washington Post* and *Wall Street Journal* of late 1975 and early 1976.
8. I. J. Selikoff, "Cancer Risk of Asbestos Exposure," presented to Meeting on the Origins of Human Cancer, Cold Spring Harbor Laboratory, New York, September 7–14, 1976; National Academy of Sciences, *Asbestos: The Need for and Feasibility of Air Pollution Controls* (Washington, D.C.: 1971); *Washington Post*, December 10, 1975.
9. Henry E. Sigerist, *Civilization and Disease* (Ithaca: Cornell University Press, 1943); Fraser Brockington, *World Health*, 2nd edition (London: J. and A. Churchill, 1967); George Rosen, "Introduction," in Bernardino Ramazzini, *Diseases of Workers*, translated by Wilmer Cave Wright (New York: Hafner Publishing Co., 1964).
10. Ramazzini, *Diseases of Workers.*
11. I.T.T. Higgins, *Epidemiology of Chronic Respiratory Disease: A Literature Review* (Washington, D.C.: Environmental Protection Agency, August 1974); Ashford, *Crisis in the Workplace.*
12. Joseph K. Wagoner, "Occupational Carcinogenesis: The Two Hundred Years Since Percival Pott," *Annals of the New York Academy of*

Sciences, May 28, 1976; Irving J. Selikoff, "Nick Evelich: In Memoriam," *Journal of Current Social Issues,* Spring 1975.

13. Ashford, *Crisis in the Workplace;* Wagoner, "Occupational Carcinogenesis."
14. John M. Peters, "Perspectives," *New England Journal of Medicine,* March 18, 1976.
15. Epidemiology Branch, National Cancer Institute, *Atlas of Cancer Mortality for U.S. Counties: 1950–1969* (Bethesda: National Institutes of Health, 1975); William J. Blot and Joseph F. Fraumeni, Jr., "Geographic Patterns of Lung Cancer: Industrial Correlations," *American Journal of Epidemiology,* Vol. 103, No. 6, 1976.
16. Lorin E. Kerr, "Coal Workers and Pneumoconiosis," *Archives of Environmental Health,* April 1968; "The Miners: A Special Case?" *Lancet,* January 19, 1974.
17. National Academy of Sciences, *Man, Materials, and Environment* (Cambridge, Mass.: MIT Press, 1973); World Health Organization, "Occupational Health Programme"; Stellman and Daum, *Work Is Dangerous to Your Health;* Coal Mines Committee, *Safety and Health in Coal Mines* (Geneva: International Labor Office, 1976).
18. World Health Organization, "Occupational Health Programme"; Pan American Health Organization, *Seminario Regional de Silicosis* (Washington, D.C.: 1970).
19. Ashford, *Crisis in the Workplace;* J. A. Fuentes, "The Need for Effective and Comprehensive Planning for Migrant Workers," *American Journal of Public Health,* January 1974.
20. Joel Swartz, "Poisoning Farmworkers," *Environment,* June 1975; Louis A. Falcon and Ray F. Smith, *Guidelines for Integrated Control of Cotton Insect Pests* (Rome: Food and Agriculture Organization, October 1973); World Health Organization, "Occupational Health Programme."
21. Kevin P. Shea, "Profile of a Deadly Pesticide," *Environment,* January/February 1977.
22. Two examples of consumer poisonings are reported in N. A. Nagi and A. K. Yassin, "Organic Mercury Poisoning in Children," *Journal of Tropical Medicine and Hygiene,* June 1974; and J. F. Copplestone, "Assignment Report on the Control of Pesticides in Sri Lanka," WHO Regional Office for South-East Asia, New Delhi, August 22, 1973.
23. On the contamination of food and the evolution of malaria resistance in Central America, see Central American Research Institute for Industry (ICAITI), *An Environmental and Economic Study of the Consequences of Pesticide Use in Central American Cotton Production* (Guatemala: ICAITI, January 1976). See also David Pimentel, "Environmental Aspects of World Pest Control," presented to Annual Meeting of the American Association for the Advancement of Science, Denver, February 20–25, 1977.
24. Morris M. Joselow, "Occupational Health in the U.S.—The Next Decades," *American Journal of Public Health,* Vol. 63, No. 11, 1973.
25. Sheldon W. Samuels, testimony before Subcommittee on Labor—Health, Education, and Welfare, Committee on Appropriations, U. S. House of Representatives, April 7, 1976.

26. Selikoff, "Nick Evelich."
27. World Health Organization, "Occupational Health Programme."
28. Madbuli Noweir, "Safe Level Criteria for Air Contaminants for Developing Countries," *Bulletin of the High Institute of Public Health of Alexandria*, Vol. V, No. 1, 1975.
29. M. A. El Batawi, "The Forgotten Masses," *World Health*, July–August 1974.
30. Useful recent reviews of women's health issues include: Phyllis Lehmann, "Women Workers: Are They Special?" *Job Safety and Health*, April 1975; Andrea M. Hricko and Cora Bagley Marrett, "Women's Occupational Health: The Rise and Fall of a Research Issue," and Jeanne M. Stellman, "Health Effects and Job Security," papers presented at AAAS Annual Meeting, New York, January 26–31, 1975; and Eula Bingham, ed., *Proceedings: Conference on Women and the Workplace* (Washington, DC.: Society for Occupational and Environmental Health, 1977).
31. Barry Castleman, a U.S. consultant, proposes the establishment of a global information system on the locations of dangerous industries in "Information Service on Worldwide Movements of Hazardous Industries," mimeo., November 9, 1976.
32. Barry Commoner, "Workplace Burden," *Environment*, July/August 1973.

Chapter 9. Of Snails and Men

1. Kathleen Courrier wrote portions of this chapter.
2. Farooq, "Historical Development," in N. Ansari, ed., *Epidemiology and Control of Schistosomiasis* (Baltimore: University Park Press, 1973).
3. G. Webbe, "Control of Schistosomiasis in Ethiopia, Sudan, and East and West African Countries," in Max J. Miller, ed., *Proceedings of a Symposium on the Future of Schistosomiasis Control* (New Orleans: Tulane University, 1972). W. H. Wright, "Geographical Distribution of Schistosomes and their Intermediate Hosts," in Ansari, *Epidemiology and Control of Schistosomiasis*, provides a global overview of schistosomiasis incidence.
4. The parasite's life cycle is reviewed in Kenneth S. Warren, "Precarious Odyssey of an Unconquered Parasite," *Natural History*, May 1974, and in Peter Jordan and Gerald Webbe, *Human Schistosomiasis* (Springfield, Ill.: Charles C. Thomas, 1969).
5. *Measurement of the Public Health Importance of Bilharziasis* (Geneva: World Health Organization, 1967).
6. "Report of the Subcommittee on Chemotherapy of Human Schistosomiasis," International Conference on Schistosomiasis, Cairo, October 18–25, 1975.
7. "Recommendations of the Subcommittee on Ecological and Habitat Control," International Conference on Schistosomiasis, Cairo, October 18–25, 1975.
8. Nelson G. Hairston, *et al.*, "Non-Chemical Methods of Snail Control," (Geneva: World Health Organization, 1975).

9. "Report of UNEP Expert Committee on Ecological and Habitat Management of Schistosomiasis" (Nairobi: United Nations Environment Program, August 1975).

10. William R. Jobin, *et al.*, "Control of Schistosomiasis in Guyana and Arroyo, Puerto Rico," *Bulletin of the World Health Organization*, Vol. 42, 1970, p. 151.

11. Joshua S. Horn, *Away with All Pests* (New York: Monthly Review Press, 1969); Mostafa Tolba, "The State of the Environment 1976," Report of the Executive Director, United Nations Environment Program, Nairobi, January 30, 1976.

12. "Country Profile: Egypt," International Conference on Schistosomiasis, Cairo, October 18–25, 1975.

13. *Schistosomiasis Control* (Geneva: World Health Organization, 1973).

14. B. B. Waddy, "Research into the Health Problems of Manmade Lakes, with Special Reference to Africa," *Transactions of the Royal Society of Tropical Medicine and Hygiene*, Vol. 69, No. 1, 1975. The potential health consequences of water resource developments are also reviewed briefly in Jane Stein, *Water: Life or Death* (Washington, D.C.: International Institute for Environment and Development, 1977).

15. Patricia Rosenfield, *Schistosomiasis Transmission Model* (Washington, D.C.: Agency for International Development, November 1975).

Chapter 10. *The Family Planning Factor*

1. Many of the topics covered in this chapter are discussed in similar terms in *The Sisterhood of Man* (New York: W. W. Norton, forthcoming), by my colleagues Kathleen Newland and Patricia McGrath. I wish to thank Kathleen Newland for her help in preparing portions of this chapter.

2. Dorothy Nortman, "Parental Age as a Factor in Pregnancy Outcome and Child Development," *Reports on Population/Family Planning*, August 1974; Abdel R. Omran, *The Health Theme in Family Planning* (Chapel Hill: University of North Carolina Population Center, 1971); Joe D. Wray, "Population Pressure on Families: Family Size and Child Spacing," in *Rapid Population Growth: Consequences and Policy Implications*, Vol. 2 (Baltimore: Johns Hopkins Press, 1971).

3. Phyllis T. Piotrow, "Mothers Too Soon," *Draper World Population Fund Report*, Autumn 1975; Frank F. Furstenburg, Jr., "The Social Consequences of Teenage Parenthood," *Family Planning Perspectives*, July/August 1976.

4. Ruth R. Puffer and Carlos V. Serrano, *Birthweight, Maternal Age, and Birth Order: Three Important Determinants in Infant Mortality* (Washington, D. C.: Pan American Health Organization, 1975).

5. Sattareh Farman-Farmaian, "Early Marriage and Pregnancy in Traditional Islamic Society," *Draper World Population Fund Report*, Autumn 1975.

6. William Burr Hunt II, "Adolescent Fertility—Risks and Consequences," *Population Reports*, July 1976.

7. Zero Population Growth, "Teenage Pregnancy: A Major Problem for Minors," Washington, D. C., March 1976; Wendy H. Baldwin, "Adoles-

cent Pregnancy and Childbearing—Growing Concerns for Americans," *Population Bulletin,* September 1976.

8. Division of Vital Statistics, U. S. Department of Health, Education, and Welfare; Robert Buchanan, "Effects of Childbearing on Maternal Health," *Population Reports,* November 1975.

9. Nicholas H. Wright, "Thailand: Estimates of the Potential Impact of Family Planning on Maternal and Infant Mortality," *Journal of the Medical Association of Thailand,* April 1975.

10. Nortman, "Parental Age as a Factor in Pregnancy Outcome and Child Development."

11. Carl E. Taylor, Jeanne S. Newman, and Narindar U. Kelly, "Interactions Between Health and Population," *Studies in Family Planning,* April 1976; Buchanan, "Effects of Childbearing on Maternal Health."

12. Dorothy E. Speed, "Population Crisis in Central Africa, Rwanda and Burundi," in G. Clifford Gould, ed., *Health and Disease in Africa—the Community Approach* (Kampala, Nairobi, Dar es Salaam: East African Literature Bureau, 1971).

13. Frank W. Lowenstein, "Some Considerations of Biological Adaptation by Aboriginal Men to the Tropical Rain Forest," in Betty J. Meggers, *et al.,* eds., *Tropical Forest Ecosystems in Africa and South America: A Comparative Review* (Washington, D. C.: Smithsonian Institution Press, 1973); K. V. Rao and C. Gopalan, "Nutrition and Family Size," *Journal of Nutrition and Dietetics,* Vol. 6, 1969, p. 258; Joe D. Wray and Alfredo Aguirre, "Protein-Calorie Malnutrition in Candelaria, Colombia. I. Prevalence; Social and Demographic Causal Factors," *Journal of Tropical Pediatrics,* September 1969.

14. J. E. Gordon, *et al.,* "The Second Year Death Rate in Less Developed Countries," *American Journal of Medical Sciences,* September 1967; D. Wolfers and S. Scrimshaw, "Child Survival and Intervals Between Pregnancies in Guayaquil, Ecuador," *Population Studies,* Vol. 29, 1975, p. 479.

15. Cicely D. Williams, "The Story of Kwashiorkor," *Courrier of the International Children's Centre,* June 1963.

16. Guillermo Arroyave, "Nutrition in Pregnancy in Central America and Panama" and David Rush, "Maternal Nutrition During Pregnancy in Industrialized Countries," in *Malnutrition and Infection During Pregnancy* (Washington, D. C.: Agency for International Development, 1975); National Academy of Sciences, *Recommended Dietary Allowances* (Washington, D.C.: 1974).

17. Derrick B. Jelliffe, *The Assessment of the Nutritional Status of the Community* (Geneva: World Health Organization, 1966).

18. J. Joseph Speidel and Margaret F. McCann, "Mini-Laparotomy—A Fertility Control Technology of Increasing Importance," presented to Association of Planned Parenthood Physicians, 14th Annual Meeting, Miami Beach, Florida, November 11–12, 1976; John Robbins, "Unmet Needs in Family Planning," *Family Planning Perspectives,* Fall 1973; Christopher Tietze, John Bongaarts, and Bruce Shearer, "Mortality Associated with the Control of Fertility," *Family Planning Perspectives,* January/February 1976.

19. Lester R. Brown and Kathleen Newland, "Abortion Liberalization: A

Worldwide Trend," Worldwatch Institute, Washington, D. C., February 1976; Margot Zimmerman, "Abortion Law and Practice—A Status Report," *Population Reports*, March 1976.

20. "Abortion: Cost of Illegality," *People* (London), Vol. 3, No. 3, 1976; Benjamin Viel, "The Sequelae of Nonhospital Abortions," in Robert E. Hall, ed., *Abortion in a Changing World*, Vol. 1 (New York: Columbia University Press, 1970); Wray and Aguirre, "Protein-Calorie Malnutrition in Candelaria, Colombia"; Leon Parrish Fox, "Abortion Deaths in California," *American Journal of Obstetrics and Gynecology*, July 1, 1967.

21. Nicholas H. Wright, "Restricting Legal Abortion: Some Maternal and Child Health Effects in Romania," *American Journal of Obstetrics and Gynecology*, January 15, 1975; *World Health Statistics Annual, 1972.* (Geneva: World Health Organization, 1975).

22. Tietze, Bongaarts, and Shearer, "Mortality Associated with the Control of Fertility"; Anrudh K. Jain, "Mortality Risk Associated with the Use of Oral Contraceptives," *Studies in Family Planning*, March 1977.

23. Richard C. Theuer, "Effect of Oral Contraceptive Agents on Vitamin and Mineral Needs: A Review," *Journal of Reproductive Medicine*, January 1972; National Academy of Sciences, "Oral Contraceptives and Nutrition," Washington, D. C., 1975; Linda Atkinson, *et al.*, "Oral Contraception: Considerations of Safety in Nonclinical Distribution," *Studies in Family Planning*, August 1974.

24. Tietze, Bongaarts, and Shearer, "Mortality Associated with the Control of Fertility."

25. Andrew P. Haynal, "Death Risk of Pregnancy and Family Planning Practice," U. S. Agency for International Development, Islamabad, May 3, 1976.

26. J. I. Mann, W. H. W. Inman, and M. Thorogood, "Oral Contraceptive Use in Older Women and Fatal Myocardial Infarction," *British Medical Journal*, August 21, 1976; Valerie Beral, "Cardiovascular-Disease Mortality Trends and Oral-Contraceptive Use in Young Women," *Lancet*, November 13, 1976; Jain, "Mortality Risk"; E. Truman Mays, *et al.*, "Focal Nodular Hyperplasia of the Liver," *American Journal of Clinical Pathology*, June 1974; Christopher Tietze, "New Estimates of Mortality Associated with Fertility Control," *Family Planning Perspectives*, March/April 1977. A report published as this book went to press suggested that, among women with a precancerous cervical condition called dysplasia, the use of oral contraceptives may increase the risk of cervical cancer. See E. Stern, *et al.*, "Steroid Contraceptive Use and Cervical Dysplasia: Increased Risk of Progression," *Science*, June 24, 1977.

27. Tietze, Bongaarts, and Shearer, "Mortality Associated with the Control of Fertility."

28. Nortman, "Parental Age as a Factor in Pregnancy Outcome and Child Development."

29. Nicholas H. Wright, "Some Aspects of the Potential Reduction in the United States Infant Mortality Rate by Family Planning," *American Journal of Public Health*, August 1972; Wright, "Thailand."

30. Speed, "Population Crisis in Central Africa"; C. Gopalan and A. N. Naidu, "Nutrition and Fertility," *Lancet*, November 18, 1972.

31. R. O. Greep, M. A. Koblinsky, and F. S. Jaffe, *Reproduction and Human Welfare: A Challenge to Research* (Cambridge, Mass.: MIT Press, 1976). This report is summarized in *BioScience,* November 1976.
32. Phyllis T. Piotrow, *World Population Crisis: The United States Response* (New York: Praeger, 1973).

Chapter 11. Creating Better Health

1. Dobzhansky quoted by René Dubos in *Man Adapting* (New Haven: Yale University Press, 1965).
2. John Bryant, *Health and the Developing World* (Ithaca: Cornell University Press, 1969).
3. Lalit Thapalyal, "Source of Life," *World Health,* July 1976.
4. World Health Organization, "Community Water Supply and Wastewater Disposal (Mid-Decade Progress Report)," Report by the Director-General, Geneva, May 6, 1976. These figures exclude China.
5. Erik P. Eckholm, *Losing Ground: Environmental Stress and World Food Prospects* (New York: W. W. Norton, 1976); Lester R. Brown, *World Population Trends: Signs of Hope, Signs of Stress* (Washington, D.C.: Worldwatch Paper 8, October 1976).
6. Bruce Stokes, *Filling the Family Planning Gap* (Washington, D.C.: Worldwatch Paper 12, May 1977).
7. I have borrowed the concept of "barefoot water-engineers" from Ian Burton and Anne Whyte, "A Choice-Benefit Approach as an Alternative to Delivery-Standard Systems in Rural Water Supply and Sanitation," mimeo, n.d.
8. Council on Wage and Price Stability, "The Problem of Rising Health Care Costs," Washington, D.C., April 1976; Conrad Taeuber, "If Nobody Died of Cancer," *Kennedy Institute Quarterly Report,* Summer 1976. For interesting perspectives on the role of medical care see John Powles, "On the Limitations of Modern Medicine," *Science, Medicine and Man,* Vol. 1, 1973, p. 1; and Warren Winkelstein, Jr., "Epidemiological Considerations Underlying the Allocation of Health and Disease Care Resources," *International Journal of Epidemiology,* Vol. 1, No. 1, 1972.
9. Marvin M. Kristein, Charles B. Arnold, and Ernst L. Wynder, "Health Economics and Preventive Care," *Science,* February 4, 1977. See also John H. Knowles, "The Responsibility of the Individual," *Daedalus,* Winter 1977, for an excellent review of the health importance of personal habits.
10. Nedra B. Belloc and Lester Breslow, "Relationship of Physical Health Status and Health Practices," *Preventive Medicine,* Vol. 1, 1972, p. 409; Nedra B. Belloc, "Relation of Health Practices and Mortality," *Preventive Medicine,* Vol. 2, 1973, p. 67.
11. Knowles, "The Responsibility of the Individual."
12. H. Mahler, "Health for All by the Year 2000," *WHO Chronicle,* December 1975.
13. Norman Gall, "The Rise of Brazil," *Commentary,* January 1977.
14. Walter Leser, "Crescimento da População e Nível de Saúde na Cidade de São Paulo," *Problemas Brasileiros,* October 1974. See also J. Yunes

and U. S. C. Ronchezel, "Evolução da Mortalidade Geral, Infantile e Proporcional no Brazil," *Revista de Saúde Publica*, for an analysis of worsening health conditions in parts of Brazil.

15. International Labour Office, *Employment, Growth and Basic Needs: A One-World Problem* (New York: Praeger, 1977), provides a useful discussion of the "basic needs" approach to development in both poor and rich countries. See also Mahbub ul Haq, *The Poverty Curtain: Choices for the Third World* (New York: Columbia University Press, 1976).

16. George M. Woodwell, "The Limits of Impoverishment: A Great New Issue," presented to AAAS Symposium on Endangered Species, San Francisco, February 28, 1974.

17. Dubos, *Man Adapting.*

18. National Academy of Sciences, *Early Action on the Global Environmental Monitoring System* (Washington, D. C.: 1976).

Suggested Readings

Ansari, N., ed. *Epidemiology and Control of Schistosomiasis (Bilharziasis)*. Baltimore: University Park Press, 1973.

Ashford, Nicholas. *Crisis in the Workplace*. Cambridge, Mass.: MIT Press, 1976.

Berg, Alan. *The Nutrition Factor*. Washington, D. C.: Brookings Institution, 1973.

Brockington, Fraser. *World Health*, Third Edition. London: Churchill Livingstone, 1975.

Bryant, John. *Health and the Developing World*. Ithaca: Cornell University Press, 1969.

Department of Health and Social Security. *Diet and Coronary Heart Disease*. London: Her Majesty's Stationary Office, 1974.

Dubos, René. *Man Adapting*. New Haven: Yale University Press, 1965.

Dubos, René. *Mirage of Health*. New York: Harper and Row, 1959.

Fraumeni, Jr., Joseph F. jed., *Persons at High Risk of Cancer*. New York: Academic Press, 1975.

Glasser, Ronald. *The Greatest Battle*. New York: Random House, 1976.

International Labour Office. *Employment, Growth and Basic Needs: A One-World Problem*. New York: Praeger Publishers, 1977.

Le Riche, W. Harding and Jean Milner. *Epidemiology as Medical Ecology*. London: Churchill Livingstone, 1971.

May, Jacques M. *Ecology of Human Disease*. New York: M.D. Publications, 1958.

May, Jacques M. *Studies in Disease Ecology*. New York: Hafner, 1961.

McKee, William D., ed. *Environmental Problems in Medicine*. Springfield, Ill.: Charles C. Thomas, 1974.

McKeown, Thomas. *The Modern Rise of Population*. New York: Academic Press, 1976.

McNeill, William H. *Plagues and Peoples*. Garden City, New York: Anchor Press/Doubleday, 1976.

Morley, David. *Paediatric Priorities in the Developing World*. London: Butterworths, 1973.

National Board of Health and Welfare. *Diet and Exercise*. Stockholm: 1972.

Newell, Kenneth W., ed. *Health by the People*. Geneva: World Health Organization, 1975.

Puffer, Ruth Rice and Carlos V. Serrano. *Patterns of Mortality in Childhood.* Washington, D. C.: Pan American Health Organization, 1973.

Saffiotti, Umberto and Joseph K. Wagoner, eds. *Occupational Carcinogenesis,* entire issue of *Annals of the New York Academy of Sciences,* May 28, 1976.

Scrimshaw, Nevin S., Carl E. Taylor, and John E. Gordon. *Interactions of Nutrition and Infection.* Geneva: World Health Organization, 1968.

United Nations, Department of Economic and Social Affairs, *Poverty, Unemployment and Development Policy: A Case Study of Selected Issues with Reference to Kerala.* New York, 1975.

Wain, Harry. *A History of Preventive Medicine.* Springfield, Ill.: Charles C. Thomas, 1970.

Warford, Jeremy J. and Robert J. Saunders. *Village Water Supply: Economics and Policy in the Developing World.* Baltimore: Johns Hopkins Press, 1976.

White, Gilbert F., David J. Bradley, and Anne U. White. *Drawers of Water.* Chicago: University of Chicago Press, 1972.

Wolman, Abel. *Water, Health and Society.* Bloomington: Indiana University Press, 1969.

World Bank. *Health: Sector Policy Paper.* Washington, D. C., March 1975.

World Health Organization. *Health Hazards of the Human Environment.* Geneva, 1972.

Index

Abortion, 192, 196–200
  availability of, 204–5, 212
  liberal laws on, 197–98
Accidents, 11, 26
Acropolis (Athens), 198
Advertising, Age of, 216
Affluence, 11, 18, 37, 209
  diets of, 62–88
  hazards of, 209
AFL-CIO, Industrial Union Division of, 168
Aflatoxin and cancer, 101
Africa
  affluent diet in, 63
  automobiles and class in, 152–53
  breastfeeding in, 50, 59
  cancer in, 79
  chemical carcinogens in, 108
  childbearing in, 195
  esophageal cancer in, 100
  fertility in, 194
  infectious diseases in, 29–31
  irrigation problems in, 186–87
  life expectancy in, 26
  nutrition education in, 59
  occupational problems in, 169
  pesticide poisonings in, 167
  pollution control in, 37, 152
  schistosomiasis in, 175–76, 180
  smoking trends in, 117–18, 123–24
  undernutrition in, 44–46
  water supply in, 29–31
Aga Khan, 67
Agricola, Georgius, 160
Agricultural extension agents, 213
Agricultural Research Service (U.S.), 126–27
Air pollution, 133–53
  from auto emissions, 136–37
  constituents of, 134, 136–38, 140–42, 144–51, 155, 158–66
  elimination of, 217
  from industry, 34–35, 134–36, 138–39, 152

  from stationary sources, 137
  See also Carcinogens
Alcoholism, 11, 34
  lifestyle and, 215
  See also Drinking
American Cancer Society, 97, 119
American Health Foundation, 97
American Heart Association, 74
American Medical Association, 73
Amniocentesis, 193
Andes Mountains, 45
Anemia, 43
  Birth control pill and, 199
Angina pectoris, 71
Ankara, (Turkey), 136
Agrentina, meat consumption in, 64
Arsenic, 145, 157–58
Asbestos
  in air, 137–38
  cancer causes in workers by, 17, 36, 159
Arterial degeneration, 18, 69–70; see also Artherosclerosis; Cardiovascular diseases
Artificial kidneys, 213
Ashford, Nicholas A., 154
Asia
  affluent diet in, 63
  automobiles in, 152–53
  breastfeeding in, 59, 195
  chemical carcinogens in, 108
  degenerative diseases in, 32–33
  fertility in, 194–95
  infectious diseases in, 30
  irrigation problems in, 186–87
  life expectancy in, 22, 26
  malaria in, 30
  occupational problems in, 169
  pesticide poisonings in, 167
  pollution control in, 37, 152
  smoking trends in, 117–18, 124–27
  undernutrition in, 41, 44–46
  water supply in, 29
Asthma, 141–42
Aswan High Dam (Egypt), 175, 187

Athens (Greece), 148
Atherosclerosis, 72–74, 87, 120
Australia
    meat consumption in, 64
    sugar consumption in, 65
Automobile pollutants, 136–37, 148–53
    health priority on, 207, 217
Automobiles
    accidents in, 25, 192
    national prosperity and, 152–53

Bacall, Lauren, 116–17
Bahamas, hypertension in, 75–76
Bangladesh
    life expectancy in, 21–22
    maternal risk with age in, 192–93
    undernutrition in, 44
Barefoot doctors, 212–13
Beer, calories in, 69
Béhar, Moisés, 49
Belgium, air pollution in, 140
Belloc, Nedra B., 215–16
Berg, Alan, 12, 23, 55, 59
Berg, John W., 12, 82
Bicycles, 207
Bilharz, Theodor, 175
Biosphere, resource management of, 7
Birch, Herbert G., 47
Birth
    age periods of safety for, 189–90, 202
    by old women, 192–93
    rate reduction of, 203
    risks of, 193–95, 202, 206
    by teenagers, 190–92, 203–4
    undernutrition and, 194
Birth control, methods of, 196–204
Birth defects among workers, 171–72
Black-lung disease, 163–64
Blindness, diabetes and, 77
Blood-fluke (parasite of schistosomiasis),
    174–81
    control of, 184
Blot, William J., 163
Bogart, Humphrey, 116–17
Bolivia
    abortions in, 197
    breastfeeding in, 220
    life expectancy in, 23
    Ministry of Public Health of, 197
    silicosis in, 164
Brazil
    General Motors in, 148
    hypertension in, 75
    income disparities in, 219
    infant mortality in, 191, 219–20
    schistosomiasis in, 176
    soybean production in, 55, 88, 219
    tobacco industry in, 125
Breastfeeding
    in Bolivia, 220
    importance of research and education
        on, 59–61
    obesity and, 68–69
    undernutrition and, 159–60
    weaning and, 40, 48, 50, 60–61
Breeder reactors, 104
Breslow, Lester, 215–16

British-American Tobacco Company, 125
Bronchitis, 25, 34, 141
Bucharest (Romania), 205
Burkitt's lymphoma, 93
Burma, workers' health in, 170

Cadmium poisoning, 35, 149
Cahill, George, 78
Cairns, John, 95, 111
Cairo (Egypt), 113, 175
Calcutta, (India), 139, 155
Cali (Columbia), 197, 210
California
    abortion complications in, 197
    State Department of Public Health in,
        165
    teenage births in, 191
Cambodia, 127
Canada
    life expectancy in, 24
    meat consumption in, 64
Cancer
    affluent diet and, 79–83, 87
    aflatoxin and, 101
    in asbestos workers, 17, 36, 98, 107
    bladder, 119
    breast, 81, 87, 93
    causes of, 18, 32–36, 90–112, 134–66
    colon, 79–81, 87
    control of, 7
    curative systems for, 213
    in developed countries, 26
    dietary fats linked to, 66, 79
    dietary influences on, 87, 101–2, 215
    from drugs, 105–7
    "endocrine-dependent" group and,
        81–82
    environmental causes of, 32–35, 91–
        112
    of esophagus, 99–100, 119
    in ideal society, 207
    larnyx, 100
    liver, 162
    lung, 33, 94–97, 117–19, 141, 144–46, 149,
        157, 162–63
    malignancies of, 89
    oral cavity, 100, 119
    pancreas, 119
    from radiation, 33, 102–5
    research of, 89–96, 99–104, 107, 110,
        181
    scrotum, 161
    stomach, 98–99. 147
    viruses and, 93
    among women workers, 171
Carbon dioxide in the atmosphere, 147
Carbon monoxide, 120–21, 131, 136–37, 140,
    144, 151
Carcinogens, 17, 32–36, 90–112
    in food, 97–99
    identified in the environment, 90–92,
        107, 109–111
    See also Cancer
Cardiovascular diseases
    affluent diet and, 78–79, 83
    birth control pill and, 199
    in contraception, 201

in developed countries, 26
in ideal society, 207–8
life expectancy and, 69–74, 77
middle-aged and, 19, 32–33
See also Arterial degeneration; Heart
disease; Stroke
Caribbean islands
life expectancy in, 22
schistosomiasis in, 176
undernutrition in, 45
Carpathian Mountains, 160
Carson, Rachel, 167
Catalytic converters, 151
Central America
pesticide effects in, 167
undernutrition in, 45
Central Asia, esophageal cancer in, 99
Charles II, 134
Chemicals, control of toxicity of, 7, 209,
217–18; *see also individual chemicals;*
Heavy metals
Chesapeake Bay, 158
Chicago (Ill.), 151
Chickenpox, 48
Chile
impaired learning ability in, 53
stomach cancer in, 99
China, 41
"barefoot doctors" of, 212–13
coronary heart disease in, 99
esophageal cancer in, 113
life expectancy in, 22
marital age in, 204
schistosomiasis in, 177, 184–86
sewage disposal in, 29
smoking in, 113
tobacco industry in, 124–26
undernourishment in, 44
water supply in, 28–29
Cholera, 29–30
Cholestrol
elevated levels of blood, 71–73
food containing, 73–74
Cigarettes, *see* Smoking
Cincinnati (Ohio), 139
Circulatory diseases, 77, 208
Cirrhosis, 34, 100–1
Ciudad Juárez (Mexico), 138
Cleveland (Ohio), 121
Coal, pollution from, 134–35, 137, 150,
163
Coal Mine and Safety Act, 164
Colombia
abortion complications in, 197
maternal mortality in, 212
poisoned by Phosvel, 166
respiratory infections in, 143–44
stomach cancer in, 99
Commodity safety, 207
Common cold, 25, 141
Commoner, Barry, 172
Congo, 194
Connecticut, ozone levels in, 138
Contraception
abortion vs., 196, 198
availability of, 204, 212
safety research on, 204

by various types, 198–201
See also Family planning
Costa Rica, sugar consumption in, 65
Counter-Blaste to Tobacco (James I),
114–15
Critchfield, Richard, 185
Cuba
life expectancy in, 23–24
sugar consumption in, 65

Dahl, Lewis K., 75–76
Dakar (Senegal), diabetes in, 77
DDT, malaria eliminated by, 26, 30–31
Death
from diarrhea, 49
prematurity of, 19, 49–51
See also Mortality
Deforestation, 134, 147
Degenerative diseases, 32–34
Detroit (Mich.) 139, 189
Diabetes, 34, 66, 68, 71, 77–78, 201
Diarrhea, 17–18, 29
in developed countries, 48–49
in developing countries, 49–50
Dickens, Charles, 135, 219
Diet, 11
of the affluent, 18, 35, 62–88, 215
basic practices of, 215
cardiovascular disease and, 33
changes from affluent, 85–88
fat in, 66, 79–83, 85
fiber in, 79–81
food additives in, 82–83
heart disease and, 33
improvement of, 135
lifestyle and, 35, 72
of the poor, 19
priorities of, 58, 207
-related cancers, 101–2
supplements for pregnancy, 59–60, 195,
206
Diets for reducing, 69
Diptheria, 207
Disease
causes vs. treatment of, 11, 209
reduction of, 206–7
from industrial causes, 35–36, 104–5,
109, 133–53, 155–72
lifestyle and, 34
spread of, 25–35
See also individual diseases
Diseases of Workers (Ramazzini), 160
Diverticulosis, 66
Dobzhansky, Theodosius, 208
Doll, Sir Richard, 103
Donora (Pa.), air pollution in, 140
Down's syndrome, 193
Drinking, 19, 34
avoidance of heavy, 207
cancer caused by, 100–1
coronary death rate and, 71
Dubos, René, 12, 221
Dysentery, 25

Eastern Europe, health hazards in, 167
Ecology of poverty, 210
Ecosystems, safeguards of, 7, 221

Ecuador, 17
  birth frequency in, 195
  fatality rate from measles, 48
Edsall, John T., 146
Education
  human needs for, 8
  in nutrition planning, 58–59
Edward I, 134
EEC (European Economic Community)
  European Commission of, 84
  tobacco subsidy provided by, 127
Egypt
  bladder cancer in, 180–81
  cotton dusts in, 20
  poisoned by Phosvel, 166
  schistosomiasis in, 18, 174–77, 180–81, 185
  tobacco under "Food for Peace" for, 127
El Batawi, M. A., 170
El Paso (Texas), 138
El Salvador, 20
  abortions in, 197
  malaria in, 167
El Salvador Maternity Hospital, 197
Elizabeth I, 114
Emphysema, 34, 141–42
Engels, Friedrich, 219
England
  cancer from smoking in, 117–18
  respiratory diseases in, 143
  smoking in, 114–16
  stomach cancer in, 99
Environment
  alteration of, 220–21
  developing countries and, 8–9
  health affected by, 7, 18–20, 33–35, 208, 218
  management of, 7–8
Environmental Protection Agency (U.S.), 108, 143
Epstein, Samuel, 126–27, 156
Esophageal cancer, 99–100
Ethiopia, 189
Eton (school, England), 115
Europe
  cancers in, 79, 100–1
  cholera in, 30
  degenerate diseases in, 32
  infectious diseases in, 25–27
  life expectancy in, 214
  maternal deaths in, 192
  meat consumption in, 64
  medical care expenses in, 214
  obesity in, 67
  overnutrition in, 34
  pesticides in, 166
  pollution control in, 37, 152
  recent development of poor countries compared with, 219
  sanitary revolution in, 211
  soybean consumption in, 57
  sugar consumption in, 65
  Thalidomide in, 106
  tobacco use in, 114–17
  urban air pollution in, 135, 138, 140, 152, 166

Evelyn, John, 134
Eye irritations, 165
Exercise
  fats and, 74
  habits of, 19, 34
  obesity and, 67–68
  priority of, 207
  See also Sedentary living

Factory workers, *see* Workers
Fallows, James, 128
Family planning, 58
  health and, 202–3, 210–12
  priorities for, 206
  research and funding of, 204–5
  See also Contraception
Famine, 38–39
Fat cells, obesity and, 68–69
Fats
  cancer and dietary, 79, 81–86, 88
  in the diet, 18, 62–66, 71–74, 216
  exercise and, 74
  unsaturated, 64, 73, 85
Fayoum (Egypt), 186
Fiber, cancer and dietary, 79–81
Filariasis, 31
Finland
  coronary mortality rates in, 72
  life expectancy in, 24
Fluorocarbons, ozone and, 146–47
Food additives
  in affluent diets, 82–83
  safety of, 207
Food programs, 58, 210
Ford Foundation, 12
  birth control study of, 204
Fossil fuels, 105, 153; *see also* Coal
Framingham (Mass.) study of coronary disease in, 71–72, 75
France
  coronary heart disease in, 70
  cuisine of, 62
  esophageal cancer in, 100
  life expectancy in, 214
  maternal mortality in, 202
  meat consumption in, 64
Fraumeni, Joseph, 107, 163

Ga (language), 195
Gastrointestinal infections, 48
General Motors, 148
Geneva, (Switzerland), 7, 204
Germany
  air pollution in, 138
  life expectancy in, 214
  occupational diseases in, 160
Ghana, schistosomiasis in, 176
Gofman, John W., 146
Gori, Gio B., 119
Great Britain
  aflatoxin in, 101
  air pollution by, 138
  cancer in, 79
  chronic bronchitis in, 141–43
  coal-burning in, 134–35
  coronary death rate in, 70
  diabetes in, 77,

Government White Paper on food pro-
    duction of, 84
Industrial Revolution in, 134–35
life expectancy in, 22
respiratory diseases in, 141–43
smoking decline in, 122
sulfur emissions in 138,
tobacco in, 126
    See also England; Scotland
Greece, fat consumption in, 64
Greece (ancient), occupational diseases
    in, 159
Guayaquil (Ecuador), 195
Guatemala
    infant diseases in, 47–48, 51
    iodized salt in, 58
    life expectancy in, 22

Haiti
    life expectancy in, 22
    undernutrition in, 45
Hawaii, bowel cancer in, 80
Haynal, Andrew P., 200
Health, defined, 8, 21
Health care, 208, 212–14, 217
Health priorities, 206–21
Health: The Family Planning Factor (au-
    thor and Newland), 13
Heart attack, 18, 25, 32, 66, 76, 214–15
    in contraception, 201
    dietary causes of, 70–72, 74–75
    in ideal society, 207
    smoking and, 119
Heart disease, 18, 32–33, 66, 68–70
    birth control pills and, 201
    causatives of, 88
    risk factors of, 71–78
    smoking and, 119
Heart failure, congestive, 75
Heavy metals
    poisoning by, 35–36
    as pollutants, 137–38, 149
Hegsted, D. Mark, 87
Henry V, 134
Herbicides, poisoning from, 165
Heredity and health, 208
Higginson, John, 110
High blood pressure, in Egypt, 181; *see
    also* Hypertension
Hippocrates
    cancer named by, 92
    dictum of, 68
Hiroshima, (Japan), 103
Hollywood (Cal.), 116–17
Hoover, Robert, 107
Hopewell (Va.), 158
Horn, Daniel, 132
Hueper, W. O., 95
Hycanthone, 181
Hyderabad (India), 194
Hydrocarbons, 136, 142, 151
Hypertension
    among air traffic controllers, 156
    among blacks, 76
    diet and, 66, 68, 71, 74–77
    lifestyles and, 215
    salt and, 75–76

Immunization, 29–30
Income, effect on health of, 23–24
India
    birth frequency in, 195
    carbon monoxide levels in, 139
    coronary heart disease in, 76
    diabetes in, 77
    night blindness in, 43
    respiratory infections in, 143–44
    tobacco in, 113, 124–25
Indian subcontinent
    life expectancy in, 23
    schistosomiasis in, 177–78
    undernourishment in, 44
    See also Bangladesh; India; Pakistan
Indonesia
    impaired child development in, 53
    poisoned by Phosvel, 166
    schistosomiasis in, 177
Industrial Revolution, 219
    air pollution in, 134–35
Industrial workers, *see* Workers
Infant diseases, 21–30, 47
Infant mortality, 22–23, 25, 27–28, 189–95,
    202–3, 209–10, 212
    in Brazil, 220
    in Guatemala, 47–48
    in Mexico, 48
    See also Life expectancy
Infectious diseases, 25–28, 135, 210–11; *see
    also specific diseases*
Influenza, 25
Insulin, 77–78
Intrauterine device (IUD), 199–200
International Agency for Research on
    Cancer (U.N.), 100
International Labor Organization, 164
International Register of Potentially
    Toxic Chemicals, 7
Ionizing radiation, 102–3
Iran, esophageal cancer in, 99–100
Israel
    schistosomiasis in, 177
    stomach cancer in, 99
    sugar consumption in, 65
Italy
    lethal chemical environment in, 34–36
    tobacco exports from, 127
Ivory Coast
    air pollution in, 148
    liver cancer in, 101

James I, 114–15
James River (Va.), 158
Japan
    cancer in, 79–81, 98–99
    coronary heart disease in, 70–71
    cuisine of, 62
    diabetes in, 78
    economic density in, 35
    hypertension in, 75–76
    Law for the Compensation of Pollu-
    tion-Related Health Damage (1973)
    of, 149–50
    life expectancy in, 214
    "manufactured" diseases in, 35
    meat consumption in, 64

monopoly of tobacco, 125
salt consumption in, 76
schistosomiasis in, 177
smoking trends in, 123
soybean consumption in, 57
sugar consumption in, 66
tobacco industry in, 125
Java, 44
Jehangir (Emperor), 115
Jelliffe, Derrick B., 196
Jinzu River (Japan), cadmium poisoning
  along, 35
Joslin Diabetes Research Center (Boston), 78

Kathmandu, 155
Kazakhstan (Soviet Union), esophageal
  cancer in, 99–100
Kenya, liver cancer in, 101
Kepone, 158–59
Kerala (Indian State), income and life expectancy in, 24
Kidney disease, 75, 77
Knowles, John H., 12, 207
Korea
  coronary heart disease in, 70
  impaired intellectual growth in children from, 54
Krokodil (Moscow magazine), 117
Kwashiorkor, defined, 42, 195

Labor unions
  environmental standards of, 172–73
  health protected by, 167–68, 170
Lagos University (Nigeria), 124
Lancet, The, 163
Laos, life expectancy in, 21–22
Latham, Michael C., 61
Latin America, 11
  automobiles in, 152–53
  breastfeeding in, 59
  chemical carcinogens in, 108
  diarrhea in, 51
  fertility in, 194–95
  infectious diseases in, 30
  irrigation problems in, 186–87
  life expectancy in, 22–23
  occupational problems in, 169
  pesticide poisonings in, 169
  pollution control in, 37, 152
  potential for cholera, 30
  smoking trends in, 117–18, 123–24
  undernutrition in, 45–46
  water supply in, 29
Lave, Lester, 148
Law for the Compensation of Pollution-Related Health Damage (1973), of Japan, 149–50
Lead poisoning, 36, 137, 140, 157
Leishmaniasis, 31
Leprosy, 31
Lesotho, 176
Leukemia, 93, 214
Libya, life expectancy in, 23
Life expectancy, 21–27
  for American males, 213–16
  for Asia, 21–25

of countries in 1970s, 21–25, 214
hypertension and, 75
overnutrition and, 45–51
practices for, 215–16
undernutrition and, 45–51
of women, 25, 216
Life Science Products, 158
Life-support systems, 220–21
Lifestyle
  air pollution and, 153
  career and, 81
  changes of, 85–86
  in developed countries, 34
  health and, 20, 24, 72, 74, 216
  hypertension and, 215
  responsible behavior and, 216–17
London (England)
  air pollution in, 36, 134–35
  chronic bronchitis in, 143
  coal-burning in, 134–37, 150,
Longevity, *see* Life expectancy
Los Angeles, 119, 139, 144, 148
  carbon monoxide concentrations in, 140
  smog in, 135–36
Lung cancer, *see* Cancer—lung

MacFarlane, Alan, 124–25
Madison Avenue, 113
Maharashtra (Indian State), 176
Mahler, Halfidan, 218
Malaria, 26, 30–32, 167, 174
Malaysia, coronary heart disease in, 70
Malnutrition, *see* Undernutrition
Manhattan (New York City), air pollution in, 138
Mao Tse-tung, 126, 177
Marasmus, 42
Massachusetts, 129–30
Massachusetts Public Health Association, 129
Maternal depletion syndrome, 196
Maternal mortality, 189
  reduction of, 202–3
Mayer, Jean, 69
McElroy, Michael, 147
Measles, 25, 48, 207
Meat
  dietary hazards of, 62–66, 74, 81–82, 86–88
  grading of, 85
  grain consumption and, 64–65, 86, 88
Medical research, 208
Medical-care systems, 11, 19–20, 212–14
  nutrition planning and, 58
  responsibility for, 217
Mediterranean region, malaria in, 30–31
Melanoma (skin cancer), 102, 147
Mercury poisoning, 138, 149
Metastasis, 92–93
Meuse Valley, air pollution in, 140
Mexico
  impaired learning ability in, 52–53
  infant mortality in, 48
  maternal mortality in, 202
  mortality of measles in, 41
  smoking trends in, 123

Mexico City, auto pollution in, 136, 152
Middle Ages, smoke pollution in, 134
Middle East
  cholera in, 30
  irrigation problems in, 186–87
  life expectancy in, 22
  schistosomiasis in, 176
  skin cancer in, 102
  tobacco industry in, 127
Minamata (Japan), mercury poisoning in, 35
Mineral deficiencies, 43
Miners, 19
  occupational diseases of, 157, 162, 163–64, 170
Minex, 158
Miridazole, 181
Miscarriages among workers, 171
Molluscicides, 182–85
Mongolism (Down's syndrome), 193
Mortality
  health care and, 209
  of infants, 22–23, 25, 27–28, 189–95, 202–3, 209–10, 220
  of mothers, 189
  rates of, 27
Moscow (USSR), smoking ban in, 130
Moses, 174
Mount Fuji, 148
Mozambique, liver cancer in, 101

Napoleon I, 175
Nasser, Lake, 176
National Academy of Sciences (U.S.), 55, 73, 147–49
  air pollution studies by, 137, 147–49
  on cholestrol and heart disease, 73
  malnutrition studies of, 55
National Cancer Institute (U.S.), 12, 103, 107, 119, 145, 157–58
  cancer survey by, 162–63
National Commission on Diabetes, 77
Near East
  smoking trends in, 124
  undernutrition in, 41
Nepal
  life expectancy in, 21–22
  tobacco in, 124–25
New England Journal of Medicine, 117
New York (State), Kepone in waters of, 158
New York City
  air pollution levels in, 138–40, 152
  hypertension in, 75
  obesity in, 68
  schistosomiasis in, 177
Nicaragua, life espectancy in, 22
Nigeria, respiratory infections in, 143–44
  smoking trends in, 123–24
Nile River, 18, 174–76, 186
Nitrogen oxides, 136, 142, 145–47, 151
Nitrosamines, 145
Nagasaki (Japan), 103
North America
  affluent diet in, 62
  air pollution in, 152
  cancers in, 79, 103

coronary heart disease in, 70
death from diarrhea in, 49
degenerative diseases in, 32
infectious diseases in, 25–27
maternal death rates in, 192
obesity in, 67
overnutrition in, 34
recent development of poor countries
  compared with, 219
sanitary revolution in, 211
sugar consumption in, 65
North Korea, 41
North Vietnam, 41
Norway
  fat consumption in, 74
  nutrition planning by, 86
Nortman, Dorothy, 202
Noweir, Madbuli, 169
Nuclear energy, 104–5, 153
Nuclear power
  exposure to radiation from, 103–4
  vs. fossil fuels, 105
Nutrition
  birth control and, 199
  health in, 189, 210
  See also Overnutrition; Undernutrition

Obesity, 66–88
  cancer and, 82
  ill effects of, 75
Occupational diseases, 154–73
  chemical sprays and, 155, 165–67
  of dye industry, 160
  of miners, 160, 163–64, 170
  of women, 170–72
  of workers, 156–58, 161–62, 170
Occupational Health and Safety Act
  (U.S.), 167–68
Oil crisis, 152–53
100,000,000 Guinea Pigs (Kallet and
  Schlink), 106
Organ transplants, 213
OPEC, 153
Overeating, *see* Overnutrition
Overnutrition, 19, 34, 37–66, 84, 215–16
  undernutrition and, 88
  See also Diet—of the affluent; Under-
    nutrition
Ozone
  deficiencies of, 146–47
  skin cancer and, 102
  in smog, 136

Page, Lot B., 76
Pakistan
  induced abortion in, 200
  life expectancy in, 22, 25
Pan American Health Organization
  (PAHO)
  childhood studies of, 45–47, 51
  smoking trends in, 123
  survey of infant deaths by, 191
Parasitic diseases, 31, 169; *see also* Schistosomiasis
Paris, (France), 66
Particulates, 148
  of radiation, 145

PCBs (polychlorinated biphenyls), 36; see
    also Pesticides
Peru, industrial pollution in, 148
Pesticides, 26, 30–31, 36–37, 165–67
Peters, John M., 162
Philadelphia
    airborne lead in, 139
    yellow fever in, 32
Philip Morris, Inc., 125
Phillipines
    coronary heart disease in, 70
    liver cancer in, 101
    maternal mortality in, 202
    protein fortification in, 58
    sugar consumption in, 66
    tobacco in, 115
Phosvel, 166
Photochemical oxidants, described, 136–
    37, 145, 151
Pittsburg (Pa.), air pollution in, 135, 140,
    150
Plutonium, 104–5, 145–46
Pneumonia, 25, 141
Poisoning
    by heavy metals, 35–36
    by lethal chemical environment, 34–36
Polio, 207
Pollution, 33
    of air, 20, 33–34, 36, 133–53
    control of, 207, 209, 217–18
    by heavy metals, 35–36, 137–38, 149
    monitoring of, 7, 221
    planned and unplanned forms of, 105
    standards of, 172
    of water, 19, 34, 47, 217
Polynesia, hypertension in, 75–76
Population control, 202
Population growth
    family planning and, 205, 211–12
    of poor countries, 219
Pregnancy
    calories needed in, 194–95
    precautions during, 206
    work during, 195–96
Protein requirements, U.N. estimate of,
    40–43
Public Law 480 (U.S.), 127
Puerto Rico
    esophageal cancer in, 100
    schistosomiasis in, 177, 186
    snail control in, 184, 186
Punjab, 195

Racoveanou, N. T., 102
Radiation
    cancer and, 102–5
    fetal exposure to, 171
Radioactive fallout, 138, 145–46, 148; see
    also Plutonium
Radithor, 106
Raleigh, Sir Walter, 114
Ramazzini, Bernardino, 113–15, 160
Record, Frank, 11, 13, 62n
Rennaisance, health problems in, 159–
    60
Respiratory diseases, incidences of, 141–
    43, 149

Richard II, 134
Rogers, Tom, 115
Romania, liberal abortion law in, 197–98
Romans (ancient)
    life expectancy of, 26
    obesity among, 67
    occupational diseases among, 159
Rosenfield, Patricia, 187
Royal College of Physicians (London),
    118
Rwanda, 203

Sahelian zone, drought in, 44
Salt, dietary hazards of, 66, 75–76, 85
Samuels, Sheldon W., 168
Sanger, Margaret, 204–5
Sanitation, 135, 189, 206–7, 209–10
    disease and, 28–29
    in Guatemala, 47–48
    schistosomiasis deterred by, 184–86
    WHO targets for 1980 on, 211
Santiago, Chile, 197
Sao Paulo (Brazil)
    air pollution in, 152
    hypertension in, 75
    infant mortality in, 191, 219–20
Sao Paulo University (Brazil), 220
Scandanavia
    air pollution in, 138
    nutrition planning in, 83–84
    workers' health protection in, 167
Schistosomiasis, 8, 31, 155
    Asian variety of, 177–78, 184–86
    carcinogenic effects of, 181
    drugs against, 181–82, 186
    in Egypt, 176–77, 180
    history of, 174–75
    prevention of, 182–84
    sanitation and, 184–85
    symptoms of, 18, 180
Scotland, cigarette smoking in, 20
Scrimshaw, Nevin S., 13, 49
Sedentary living, 19, 33, 66–68, 71–72, 85,
    215
Selikoff, Irving J., 91, 161, 168
Senegal, 77
Seskin, Eugene, 148
Seventh-Day Adventist Church, 24
    cancer studies of, 81
Seveso (Italy), poisonous chemicals over,
    36
Sewage, 211; see also Sanitation
Sharpston, Michael, 27
Shea, Kevin P., 166
Sigerist, Henry E., 160
Silicosis, 164
Singapore, 66
Smallpox, 26, 30
Smith, Adam, 220
Smog, 135–36, 217
Smoke pollutants, 34, 133–36, 217
Smoking, 19–20, 33, 100–1, 105, 109, 132,
    145, 149
    advertising and, 216
    cancer caused by, 96, 144–45
    costs of, 129–30
    in developed countries, 34